D1481731

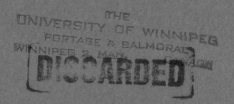

Hospital Organization

Hospital Organization

A Progress Report on the Brunel Health Services Organization Project

RALPH ROWBOTTOM
with
Jeanne Balle   Stephen Cang
Maureen Dixon   Elliott Jaques
Tim Packwood   Heather Tolliday

Distributed in the United States by
CRANE, RUSSAK & COMPANY, INC.
347 Madison Avenue
New York, New York 10017

Heinemann Educational Books Ltd
London Edinburgh Melbourne Auckland Toronto
Hong Kong Singapore Kuala Lumpur
Ibadan Nairobi Johannesburg New Delhi

ISBN 0 435 85820 3
© Ralph Rowbottom 1973
First published 1973

Published by Heinemann Educational Books Ltd
48 Charles Street, London
W1X 8AH

Printed in Great Britain by
Northumberland Press Ltd
Gateshead

Foreword

The research projects on which this book is based have both a practical and a theoretical object. The practical object has been to assist members of the health service to analyse and to understand more clearly the nature of the organizational structures best suited to the functioning of the service. It was assumed that this clarification could lead to changes in organization which might help to ensure the more effective use of the comparatively scarce resources and thus to improve the quality of the service.

The theoretical object has been to contribute to the understanding of complex organizations and of professional work. It has been assumed that the access to real social situations achieved in the course of the practical work in hospitals would make it possible to learn about this very complex type of organization with its multi-professional groups by providing the opportunity to observe at first hand how it manages to function.

The practical results achieved so far are described in this book. In addition, members of the research unit have been invited by the Department of Health and Social Security to assist in the re-organization of the health services about to be undertaken. The concepts here described are thus undergoing a stringent and practical test in that new situation, the outcome of which remains a matter for the future.

On the theoretical side, we have begun to make preliminary formulations of the reasons why different types of organizational pattern are required in the health services – to cope with the mixture of hierarchically organized work and clinical autonomy, and to take into account the amalgam of professionally-based services all brought together in the interests of the patient. Some of these preliminary formulations are presented here, and their linkages with other work are considered. But this theoretical work has only begun, and we hope during the next phase of our research to extend and deepen our theoretical formulations in conjunction with the continuing analysis of the results of our practical work.

Since this book was completed the Department of Health and Social Security have published their *Management Arrangements for the Reorganized National Health Service* (Her Majesty's Stationery Office, London, 1972) – known as the 'Grey Book'. Scrutiny of the Grey Book will make it clear how much the Brunel contribution to the formulation of these management arrangements arose from the material described in the present book.

II

The book is based upon field work carried out by present and past members of the research team. Each of us has been involved in work in at least two hospital groups, some in teaching hospitals and in medical schools, some at Regional Hospital Board level and some in the Department of Health and Social Security. And each has taken part in our training conference programmes. It is out of all this work that the concepts presented have emerged.

In order to arrange this material for publication, however, it proved necessary to designate one member of the research team to undertake the task of writing. Books cannot be written by research teams. We chose Ralph Rowbottom for this task. The book thus represents his view of our research developments, and uses many examples from his own field work. The other authors have taken part in developing the outline of the presentation and have commented in detail upon the text. We hope that this mode of presentation will thus provide a coherent account, in one person's style, of work contributed to by a number of colleagues – both those now in the research team and others who have been members in the past.

III

The work has proved exceedingly stimulating, since the whole field of health service organization is in a state of creative ferment. Our prime acknowledgment must be to Mr. J. B. Cornish and other officers of the Department of Health and Social Security, and to Mrs. A. S. Blofeld, Mr. G. H. Weston, Mr. F. J. Short, and other officers and members of the North West Metropolitan Regional Hospital Board, who initiated sponsorship for the research and have encouraged members of the health service to become actively involved. Our first work base was at the Westminster Hospital Group, and the fact that that project has become our longest continuous collaboration is due to Mr. R. P. MacMahon, Miss M. Mudge, Dr. J. B. Wyman and their colleagues in the hospital and the medical school.

From the University side special acknowledgment must be made to Maurice Kogan, now Professor of Government and Social Administration at Brunel, who as Director of the Unit (then the Hospital Organization Research Unit) in its first formative years did so much to establish its position and reputation. The authors are indebted also to the work of a number of colleagues now no longer with the Health Services Organization Research Unit, notably Maureen Cain and Robert Miller, and to two other colleagues outside the research, John Evans and David Marsland, for their frequent comments and advice.

Finally, convention apart, spontaneous gratitude demands mention of the debt to our secretarial staff. Under Lynn Drummond and Mollie Parish, they have maintained an administrative service of high efficiency, and unfailing and essential support to the research team at all times.

Elliott Jaques
October 1972

Contents

FOREWORD   v

1. Introduction – The Project and this Book   1
2. General Outline of Health Services in 1971   14

Part I. Elements of Hospital Organization

3. The Nature of Organization – An Initial Conception   25
4. Kinds of Roles and Role-Structures in Hospitals   40

Part II. Patterns of Existing Hospital Organization

5. Organization of Medical Staff   73
6. Organization of Paramedical Staff   100
7. Organization of Nursing Staff   119
8. Organization of Other Hospital Staff   148
9. The Role of Administrators and Finance Staff   172
10. Group and Regional Organization   188

Part III. Conclusions and Departures

11. Some General Conclusions from Project-Work So Far   213
12. General Implications for Organizational-Design in the
        Health Field   223
13. Some Open Issues   246
14. Retrospect and Prospect   259

APPENDIX A. Glossary   261
APPENDIX B. Social Analysis in Large-Scale Organizational
        Change   276
BIBLIOGRAPHY   301
INDEX   307

1 Introduction –
The Project and this Book

Brief History of the Project

This book is a report of an exploration in hospital organization – a report of work still in progress.

In October 1967 the then Ministry of Health[1] agreed to sponsor a unit (the Hospital Organization Research Unit)[2] in the School of Social Sciences at Brunel University to carry out work in this field. The initial sponsorship was for three years, though the period was later extended. It was understood from the beginning that the Unit would be concerned not merely with *study* but with *change*; and in consequence, that the choice of method of work would be critical. An initial team of four researchers was created, and projects were gradually started in two teachings groups – the Westminster and King's College in London – in the Redhill and Netherne Group in the South West Metropolitan Region; and later on a limited scale with a third teaching group – the Charing Cross Group – in London.

In 1968, officers of the North West Metropolitan Regional Hospital Board approached Brunel with a request for help in establishing systematic management-training and development programmes. A programme of collaboration was agreed, including the financing of a small additional research team at Brunel for an initial period of three years (again later extended). The specific job of this team was to provide a base of research and pilot development within the Region on which a comprehensive Regional structure of policy on organizational matters, together with a

[1] Since November 1968 the Department of Health and Social Security (D.H.S.S.).
[2] Now the Health Services Organization Research Unit.

closely-integrated training programme, could gradually be built.

This second team started intensive work in the Hillingdon Hospital Group (in the North West Metropolitan Region) late in 1968, and, with staff from the main Unit, additional projects were started in 1969 in the new Northwick Park Hospital and in the central organization of the North West Metropolitan Board itself. In 1970 further projects were launched in the Staines, the Central Middlesex, and the North London Hospital Groups. Inevitably, the work of the main Unit and the separately-sponsored research team became more and more intertwined, and late in 1970 they were combined as one administrative unit, having two separate sources of finance and sponsorship.

In May 1969 the first of a series of interdisciplinary conferences for senior staff of the North West Metropolitan Region was held with the dual aims, first of forwarding the process of management development by giving hospital staff the opportunity to study the emerging research findings from specific projects, and secondly, of establishing the generality of these findings by testing them against the collective experience of a wider audience. The series has continued, in events ranging from three days up to four weeks in length, at the total rate (at time of writing) of about twenty weeks per year. It has been attended by officers and staff from Regional, H.M.C. and hospital level – doctors, nurses, administrators, and senior staff from a wide range of other hospital professions.

At the time of writing, then, there is a team of about ten researchers currently engaged on intensive field-projects in half a dozen or so varied hospital sites, working at all levels from ward up to Regional Board (or Board of Governors), and, at one time or other, in virtually all departments of the service.

The Method of Work

Certain key features of the approach have been indicated above – study, collaboration, training, development. Right at the heart of the work is the idea that a close collaboration of researchers and hospital service staff in studying problems of organization and management that actually concern hospitals, will provide the best opportunities of:

(a) understanding the real nature of these problems in explicit terms;

(b) undertaking experiments in controlled change to resolve these problems;

(c) providing opportunities for training programmes intimately linked to the reality of the specific situations in which hospital staff work.

Following this principle, all project activities, both fieldwork and training, are guided by steering committees on which are represented both members of the hospital service and researchers. Overall guidance is provided by a steering committee within the Department of Health and Social Security itself, regional guidance by a steering committee within the Region chiefly concerned, and local guidance by steering committees at Group level. It is for the local steering committee (which typically includes the Chairman of the Hospital Management Committee, the Group Secretary, the Chief Nursing Officer, a senior medical representative and some-times the Treasurer) to decide which particular projects shall be undertaken and with what priority.[3] It will decide whether, for example, the prime need is to help clarify a particular area of nursing organization, or a ward housekeeping scheme, or the or-ganizational relationships of hospital chief officers; or to help with a quite small and specific problem, like the division of account-ability for the control of engineering stores. The willingness of the particular group of staff concerned to collaborate in the proposed project is then tested in a group discussion. If they do not want to collaborate there is obviously a problem, but it is a problem which rests with the steering committee as a whole, and not just with the researchers. Given the willingness of the group to join in, the next step is to hold a series of confidential discussions with each member of the group.[4] Each individual's initial assumptions about his

[3] Of the Hospital Internal Communications Project, also concerned with the promotion of organizational change, Weiland (1971) who acted as evaluator, reported that potentially the most important factor in success was the extent to which members of the hospital project-teams made their usual work a part of the project, and vice versa (page 293). Exactly the same might be said of this project. He stressed also the unlikelihood of success where significant members of the group or 'role-set' who would naturally be con-cerned with any project were not in fact involved in the project-work itself. Again the parallel is exact.

[4] It is not unusual, for example, to have in the first place from two to four discussions with each individual, each one or to two hours in length. Further discussion with the same individual might well be undertaken at a later stage.

organizational situation and problems will be elicited (the *assumed* situation), and any differences between these assumptions and how things work on paper (the *manifest* situation) or how they really tend to work in practice (the *extant* situation) will be discussed. Eventually, an agreed analysis of his situation can, with his permission, be circulated amongst his colleagues, and their agreed analyses sent to him. Group discussions then follow (at this stage confidential to the group), and a general analysis can be produced with, it is to be hoped, indications of points where changes or clarification will lead to a more workable (or *requisite*) organization.

And so the process continues. Analysed material gradually flows upwards to local steering committees, and when cleared by them to Regional or Departmental level, as the case may be. At each level, opportunities for organizational clarification or change present themselves, and the authorities concerned at each level may then, in principle, act on them.

Thus the research design is not that of a survey, or even a case study, but one which looks to a practical outcome in the form of change, in the study situation.[5] Whether this pragmatic approach reduces or enhances the theoretical value and strength of what is learned *en route*, must be left to the reader's own judgement as the material is displayed. On the other hand, it is an approach which must be distinguished from that of management consultancy. At no time are 'recommendations' made by the researcher. His particular role in this project is catalytic – it is his part to provide a continuous analytical contribution to the thinking of those who are charged with making decisions or recommendations. All administrators must in the nature of things commit themselves to decisions one way or the other as deadline approaches. So too, management consultants must commit themselves to this recommendation or that, if recommendations are what they are hired to make. But the analyst in this research is not bound by pressure of

[5] In this it is in common with the large-scale Hospital Internal Communications Project, inspired by Revans (Revans 1971, Weiland 1971), and the work of Pantall and Elliott (1968) in the East Birmingham Hospital Group. The work of Williams (1969) too, though starting from a training base, has a strong orientation to specific change in the organizational situation based on the use of in-site 'working-parties', and starting (as here) from an analysis of how 'defined' situations (as he calls them) vary from the 'extant' and 'requisite'.

needs in the same way. His endpoint is the moment when the particular organizational problem posed has been explained, analysed, and resolved to the satisfaction of all concerned – including his own. At this time, no 'recommendations' from him are needed; before this time, his work of elucidation is incomplete. (Further discussion of this method is contained in Appendix B.)

The Scope of the Work

There is an infinite variety of aspects of the life and work of hospitals which might conceivably be studied with benefit. Naturally, our work cannot study them all. We have not systematically studied, for example, the nature of the social, economic or epidemiological environment within which hospitals operate; the origin, training, characteristics, or attitudes, of various groups of staff who work in hospitals, or of their patients; the administrative methods which are employed – the specific techniques of operational research, of planning, of budgeting, of financial control, etc. We have not studied alternative systems of clinical and nursing management, of hospital layout, of central service supply, of planned preventive maintenance and so on. Many other workers have studied, and are studying, these things to effect (see Note at end of chapter).

Our work so far has concentrated on purely organizational issues – what roles particular groups and individuals play, and how these roles do (or do not) bind together as one system in forwarding the work of the hospital as a whole. Looked at another way, the work is about how decisions of various kinds are made in hospitals, who is agreed to have authority to make them, and who is therefore accountable for the outcomes. Thus we might explore with a nurse such questions as:

- exactly what functions, or duties do you consider yourself accountable for carrying out, and to whom are you accountable for the performance of these duties?
- what discretion do you have in carrying out these duties? What decisions are yours alone to make, which are the doctors', which must be agreed jointly?
- how do you see the authority of various senior nurses, doctors and administrators, with whom you interact?

– if you would wish to see changes in your own role, or in policies
which affect you, what means are open to you to initiate them?[6]

Such explorations have now been carried out in depth with some
hundreds of senior hospital staff: with doctors of all grades, with
many nurses of charge-nurse grade and upwards, as well as some
staff nurses, with Group and Hospital Secretaries and their assistants, and with heads of paramedical and service departments of
all kinds.

But where, the reader may ask, does the patient come in all this?
Study of the care actually received by the patient, and the quality
of relationships with those echelons of staff – doctors, junior nurses,
aides of various kinds – in immediate contact with patients[7] certainly seems a natural place to start, and many past studies have
been concerned with just such questions. Explicitly or implicitly
such studies often imply reviews of social policy or clinical outlook.
Inevitably the researcher finds himself to some extent in the position of critic or advocate – suggesting that more resources are
needed here or greater enlightenment of approach there. In our
research such an independent stance, appropriate though it may
be for other approaches, is neither sought nor possible. Our work
is not concerned with an independent critical evaluation of the
services received by patients. It is avowedly about how hospital
staff can be helped to organize themselves in ways which are more
effective *according to their own definitions of appropriate functions*, subject to the ultimate sanction of higher authorities. Ultimately of course such work may reasonably be expected to help

[6] Students of management may well ask at this point: are you studying
merely the *formal* organization (in the sense classically defined by Roethlisberger and Dickson (1939), or at a later date for instance by Blau and Scott
(1963))? The rapid answer is that we are trying to get out in explicit terms
the real (i.e. *extant*) role-system which people adopt in order to get the work
done, in order that we may study with them whether or not it is *requisite*.
At the same time, it is not claimed that this is the only role-system to be
discerned in the social structure of hospitals, or the only one capable of
institutionalization – see for example the discussion of representative role-
systems in Chapter 4. The language of *formal* and *informal* organization
has not been found useful in this research, and indeed in general, as Mouzelis
(1967, page 47) has well demonstrated, is shot through with inherent am-
biguities.

[7] Work exemplified, for instance, in classic studies of mental hospitals such
as those of Stanton and Schwartz (1954), and Goffman (1968).

rather than hinder the quality of service produced by hospitals,[8] but we have certainly not, at this point at any rate, attempted to establish positive evidence of any links between the two.[9]

The Type of Problems Encountered

The following are some examples of the type of problems we have encountered.

Firstly, there are problems about the organizational position of doctors. Their actions and influence certainly have a major effect on the quality of the service and on the costs incurred in hospitals, and they are often adjured to take account of their managerial role. Are doctors really managers? If so whom exactly do they manage? Given the unquestioned fact of their clinical autonomy (at least in the consultant grade) in what sense, if any, can they in turn be managed? And further, if being fully managed, in any real sense of the phrase, is incompatible with clinical autonomy (as we now believe it to be) what means exist to influence or curb their work at all?

This naturally leads to the role of medical committees. If their chairmen do not play a managerial role what in fact is their function? Is it more appropriate that they should be elected by their fellows, or appointed by the hospital authority? What happens if an individual consultant, though 'outvoted' in committee, ignores the decision and resolutely carries on in his own way?

What exactly is the organizational position of the member of paramedical staff, the radiographer, the physiotherapist, the laboratory technician? Granted that he is subject to medical direction, is he in fact *accountable* to any doctor? And if he is, how is this reconcilable with the fact that the two are commonly working for different employers, the Regional Hospital Board and the Hospital Management Committee respectively, and that the local adminis-

[8] Revans' (1964) demonstration of the correlation between quality of service (as indicated by average length of stay by patients) and the quality of internal staff relationships (as indicated by attitudes of ward sisters to both their superiors and their subordinates) provides general reinforcement to the argument here.

[9] See the discussion in Appendix B of the problems of establishing appropriate criteria for, and evidence of, the ultimate benefit of any organizational development of the kind undertaken in this project.

trator commonly also has close concern with the management of his work?

And then there is the administrator himself, caught in an increasing trend to 'functional' management with the appointment at group, area, or regional, level of senior specialists such as engineers, building officers, pharmacists and supplies officers. He sees in this situation an increasing threat to his organizational position. How far does his accountability and authority now stretch? Does he carry full managerial authority, with powers to prescribe and sanction in respect of local departmental heads, paramedical, nursing or even medical? Or is he predestined for some apparently lesser role, in which he must eternally rely on powers of tact and persuasion alone in order to see that the work of the hospital as a whole still gets done?

What is the role of chief administrator in relation to nursing, with the advent of the new central 'chief nursing officer' in place of the older federation of matrons of separate hospitals? Has he now lost all responsibility for nursing work?

And what of these new chief nursing officers themselves? How is their role different from that of the old-time matron? How many layers of nursing administrators are needed between these chief nursing officers and the work of the wards, without rendering them remote on the one hand, or overburdened with pressing detail on the other? Must all senior nursing roles be conceived in the same managerial pattern? Is there room for other kinds of role, with a complementary function? The new charge-nurse (once ward sister) moves in a new world of ever-increasing technical and organizational complexity. Once almost literally 'head cook and bottle-washer' as well as a nurse, she must now work alongside an increasing brigade of clerks, domestics, housekeepers and caterers. What is her responsibility now, for the work of these people?

And so to the hospital, and to the Hospital Group as a whole. Who *is* accountable for seeing that the whole complex works; for ensuring that beds are properly allocated, drug bills and other expenditure kept in proper balance, that all the services provided for patients are adequately assessed, and developed with a due sense of the priority of community needs; for seeing that adequate supporting services are developed and provided? Does, or could, any one officer hold this accountability, or must it rest in the end with the governing body itself – the Hospital Management Committee, or Board of Governors, for example? Is the role of such a body primarily indeed to 'manage' the hospitals, or is it to represent the consumers of services, or is it perhaps even to represent the staff? May these three roles be combined without conflict or ambiguity?

And finally to the role of higher authority itself, in relation to this governing body – for example the role of the Regional Hospital Board towards the Hospital Management Committee, or the role of the Department of Health and Social Security towards the Regional Hospital Board and the Board of Governors.[10] Is the relationship between the two simply managerial? May the higher body direct the lower at all times, and in all matters; or has the lower some residual, and inalienable 'rights'? If there is indeed real authority between the two, to what extent does this spread to the respective officers? May for example, regional engineers give straightforward instructions to group engineers, and if so in what circumstances, and with what reservations?

The Purpose of the Book

The main purpose of this book is to make an interim report of the results of field and conference work on such questions to date. So far much progress has been made on a wide front, it is believed, in understanding the nature of present hospital organization, and of perceiving the emergence of a number of detailed alternatives in various parts of the service. In order to do this it has been necessary to produce a number of new tools for the very act itself of *description* of hospital organization, for we did not feel that adequate tools were available at the start of our work. As we shall see, such conceptual or descriptive tools were not rapidly produced: they have been forged slowly and painfully over a period of time.

However, it must frankly be reported that little so far has been achieved in the way of explicitly-agreed and explicitly-tested change, though this is not to say that there may not have been many important changes in insight and attitude as a result of the work. Partly this has been due to the unexpected difficulty of the first part of the task, in understanding with sufficient clarity the enormous complexity of hospital organization as it exists at present.

[10] For details of the post-1948 structure of the hospital service see Chapter 2.

Partly it is no doubt due to the very considerable difficulty of instituting formal and explicit change in a service where this would carry national implications and thus require sanction at a considerable number of successive levels of authority.

At the moment of writing, the first batch of explicit proposals for pilot changes are in process of reaching approval at Regional and National level, and the strategies of implementation and evaluation are being planned in detail. It is hoped that the results of these pilot projects may be reported in detail in later publications as each or several come to fruition.

Thus what can be reported for the moment are largely findings of the extant situation – how hospitals are *really* organized in their various parts, as opposed to how they are often stated or thought to be organized. Sometimes a number of alternatives have to be described, either because it is clear that different patterns are employed in different project-sites; or (quite frequently) because the people in any particular project-area can see various alternatives, but cannot readily reach agreement on which pattern they either do or would like to adopt in practice so that the situation remains for them clouded.

Given the method of work and its commitment to confidentiality until the clientele concerned are satisfied that they have clarified their problem and are prepared to release details to a larger audience, it is not possible by and large to identify the particular hospitals and groups of staff concerned in the various projects to be described.[11]

The Outline of the Book

The text that follows is divided into three main parts.

Part I. Elements of Hospital Organization, starts by describing the basic organizational concepts which have been brought to the research in the first place, in order to generate description and analysis – concepts of the nature of authority and accountability, of operational work, of duties and tasks and so on. Using this

---

[11] One exception is the housekeeping project at Dulwich Hospital described in Chapter 8, details of which have already been reported publicly. Again, it is hoped as time goes on to report an increasing number of agreed pilot projects in quite specific detail as implementation proceeds.

initial framework, the next chapter describes how definitions of the various existing elements of hospital organization were slowly forged and tested in project discussion – the meaning of a managerial relationship, of the treatment-prescribing roles of doctors, of monitoring roles and co-ordinating roles, staff officer and supervisory roles, what it means to play a 'representative' role and so on. (These elements can be thought of as the basic building blocks of hospital organization, present or future.)

Part II. Patterns of Existing Hospital Organization, the results of studying and analysing the organization of various groups of staff in hospitals – nurses, doctors, administrators, paramedical staff, etc. – in terms of the organizational elements described in Part I are reported. Where discussion has revealed a number of apparent organization alternatives, these too are given; for example possible alternative structures for the organization of radiographers vis-à-vis radiologists and hospital administrators. Finally the results of study of some broader investigations – the operational functions of the present Hospital Service, the relative roles of the R.H.B. and H.M.C., and of their respective officers, are reported. All these findings are then brought together to show the general 'multi-partite' nature of the present management structure of hospitals.

Part III. Conclusions and Departures summarizes the main conclusions to be drawn from project-work so far, and discusses their immediate implications for organizational planning not only in hospitals, but in the health field generally. Some other issues of general importance, not yet by any means fully analysed in project-work, but now rapidly coming into view, are summarized as well.

In order to allow as free a flow as possible to the main narrative, factual details such as the number and kinds of people worked with in any project-area (up to the autumn of 1971) along with various broader comments and references to previous official hospital reports and to the literature in general, are taken out of the text and given in notes. For convenience of reference, the various organizational definitions scattered through Chapters 3 and 4 are gathered in one place in alphabetical order in Appendix A. Appendix B contains a rather longer excursion into the method of 'social analysis', its relationship to other methods of social study, and its role in both the production of scientific knowledge and in the bringing-about of large-scale organizational change.

Note to Chapter 1

The General Field of Hospital Research (page 5)

It may help in fixing the scope of this particular kind of project-work to relate it to the field of hospital research more generally, which may be seen as falling into the following broad categories:

(1) studies of the *techniques of hospital operation*, i.e. mostly clinical and nursing research;

(2) studies of the *goals and programmes of hospital operation* – epidemiological and econometric studies, health policy studies;

(3) studies of *hospital support activities* – hospital design, studies of manpower planning and recruitment, supplies, laundry, C.S.S.D., etc., etc.;

(4) studies of *administrative techniques* – research on planning systems, control systems, costing systems, etc.;

(5) studies of *style and attitudes* – of managerial styles used, of staff attitudes, of the quality of personal communication in hospitals, etc.; and finally,

(6) studies of *roles and role-structure*.

All these, with the exception of the first, might with some justification be described in general as studies of hospital organization or hospital management, and researchers pursuing these latter topics have moved freely across the various areas. The operational researchers have worked mainly in the second, third and fourth areas. (Cornish and MacDonald 1971.) The work of Crichton (1965) and her associates on manpower planning, for example, falls in the third. Menzies' (1960) notable paper falls in the fifth. Revans' (1964) original work on hospital morale and communication obviously fits the fifth category too, but the later work of the Hospital Internal Communication Project (Revans 1971, Weiland 1971) although starting from the fifth area (style and attitude) has moved freely into aspects of hospital management falling in a number of categories listed above. So, too, has the work of Pantall and Elliott (1968) deriving also from Revans' original studies. They report for example work on a wide variety of subjects such as staff-attitudes, management activity analysis, management-by-objective schemes, job-descriptions, staff meetings, length of stay by patient – the main defining principles being staff participation in the research, and concern for the work of the hospital as a whole.

By and large the studies of medical sociologists have been relevant mainly to the second field of interest listed above, though some of their work is directly concerned with the sixth field – role and role-structure. Reader (1963) discusses four main areas of existing medical sociological studies:

   (i) the social etiology and ecology of disease;
  (ii) social components in therapy and rehabilitation;
 (iii) medicine as a social institution;
 (iv) the sociology of medical education.

Nevertheless Cornish (1971) concludes that, for Britain at least, the part that serious research has played in the field of hospital management (sic) has until recently been small (p. 169). As far as the study of the sixth area, the role structure of hospitals is concerned, the main British contribution comes from the various official reports on hospital organization published over the years – Bradbeer (1954), Salmon (1966), Farquharson-Lang (1966) 'Cogwheel' (1967) and many others. (Note that 'role-structure' here refers to that obtaining amongst organization-members, and therefore excludes an alternative view which grants patients as well, for example, a 'sick-role' in some broader social scheme. For our purposes, patients are not part of the organization, but are, on the contrary, there to be served by it.)

Perrow (1965) in an important survey of the literature on hospital organization suggests that the vast American literature in this field falls into two main categories. The greater part is concerned with mental hospitals, carries a 'reforming zeal' and is frequently concerned with 'milieu therapy' (i.e. falls mainly into the first and fifth areas listed above). Typically, there is little emphasis on role-structure in this literature '... the needs of the people and their inter-personal relationships become the primary focus, while the objective fact of what they bring with them to the situation and the nature of the work done in the situation is de-emphasized' (p. 935). The other and lesser section of the field, that concerned with general hospitals, has for the most part, according to Perrow, been relatively trivial in content (p. 913). The main question addressed might be said to be: 'does the hospital as a form of social organization, constitute a major and significant deviation from conceptions of bureaucracy that stemmed from the analysis of governmental bureaucracies and economic organizations? Is the organization for service, utilizing independent professionals, a markedly different beast?' (p. 947).

At least Goss (1963) and Smith (1958) have had important contributions to make on this question, and it is one, as we shall see, which is very much of concern too in the project to be described overleaf.

2 General Outline of Health Services in 1971

The project-work to be described has been carried out in a hospital service whose basic structure, of course, was established as part of the National Health Service in 1948. It may, therefore, be a useful preliminary to sketch the outlines of this structure and its place within the National Health Service as a whole. Readers who are familiar with this subject will no doubt proceed to the next chapter.

It is worth noting at the outset that what can be described is, in the terms of this research, simply a 'manifest' structure. The general outlines are written in legislation and regulation, and are there for all to see; but how these outlines are interpreted in practice, and what detailed arrangements are made within them – the 'extant' organization – is a matter for just the kind of exploration with which this whole project is concerned. There is simply no straightforward answer, precise and detailed, to the question how hospital services are organized at present. There is abundant documentary evidence on the one hand; there is a wide variety of individual working assumptions on the other.

Nevertheless there would no doubt be universal agreement as to the present basic structure at least at the level of generality shown in Figure 2.1.[1]

Health services in England and Wales are administered locally in several different ways.

[1] For a more detailed description of this basic structure see Volume 1 of the Acton Society Trust (1955) Survey of hospitals under the N.H.S., or relevant sections of the Guillebaud Report (1956) which gives much useful information. More up-to-date descriptions will be found in a Central Office of Information publication 'Health Services in Britain' (1968), and in Chaplin (1969).

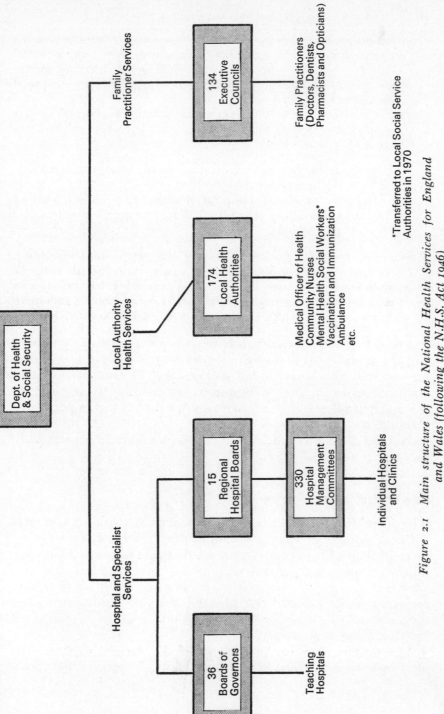

Figure 2.1 Main structure of the National Health Services for England and Wales (following the N.H.S. Act 1946)

(1) *Family Practitioner Services.* The services of family doctors ('general medical practitioners'), family dentists, and pharmacists and opticians who practise on their own in the community are provided through contracts with 134 specially-composed Executive Councils.

(2) *Hospital and Specialist Services.* Hospitals and a range of services of specialists such as medical consultants, are provided by three kinds of statutory body:

    (a) thirty-six Boards of Governors in the case of the majority of teaching hospitals;

    (b) fifteen Regional Hospital Boards with the assistance of 330 subsidiary Hospital Management Committees for other hospitals.

(3) *Local Authority Services.* Most of the other statutory health services – community nursing, vaccination, health centres, ambulances, etc. (see below) – are provided by 174 county councils, county borough councils and London borough councils. Environmental health services are provided by district councils.

The first two categories, family practitioner services and hospital and specialist services, are financed by central government except for receipts from charges for services and certain money from endowments in the case of hospitals. Local authority services, on the other hand, are financed basically from rates (again with help from receipts from charges for services) but with very substantial Exchequer help through the rate-support grant. In more detail, these parts work as follows.

Family Practitioner Services

The main function of Executive Councils is to make contracts with the various categories of family practitioner, to provide services in their area. They have to see that lists of practitioners are published and that patients receive adequate personal care and attention. In conjunction with a committee established by the Secretary of State, called the Medical Practices Committee, they must control the number of medical practitioners operating in their area under these services.

The doctors, dentists, pharmacists and opticians in each area elect their own committees, and the Council is required to consult with them in exercising its functions. Each Executive Council itself consists of thirty-five members:

- eight appointed by the local health authority;
- seven by the Secretary of State;
- eight by the Local Medical Committee (one of them an ophthalmic practitioner);
- three by the Local Dental Committee;
- two by the Local Pharmaceutical Committee;
- an ophthalmic optician appointed by ophthalmic opticians on the Local Optical Committee;
- a dispensing optician appointed by dispensing opticians on the Local Optical Committee.

Since 1949, the Committee elects its own Chairman.

Local Health Services

The health functions carried out by local authorities included until recently provision of all the following services:

(1) health care for mothers and young children (including provision of ante-natal, post-natal and infant welfare clinics, of dental care of expectant mothers and young children, and of day-nurseries);
(2) home midwifery;
(3) home nursing and health visiting;
(4) home helps;
(5) vaccination and immunisation;
(6) ambulance services;
(7) services for the mentally ill and mentally handicapped (including training centres and hostels);
(8) family planning;
(9) health education;
(10) school health services;
(11) a variety of other preventive and aftercare services;
(12) health centre facilities in certain places, for the use of family practitioners and associated local authority staff;
(13) environmental health services (e.g. food hygiene and prevention of spread of infectious diseases).

Most of these functions were formerly the responsibility of the health committees of local authorities, though provision of school health services was, and is, the responsibility of the education committee. However, following the arguments of the Seebohm Report, it was considered that some of these functions – for example provision of day nurseries and home helps, and all work with the mentally disordered – would be more suitably given to the new Social Services Departments, established under the 1970 Act.[2]

Both local health committees and local social service committees are of course sub-committees of the main local authority, and as such are wholly responsible to that body.

Regional Hospital Boards

The main functions of the fifteen Regional Hospital Boards (R.H.B.s), including the Welsh Hospital Board which is subject to the administration of the Welsh Office rather than the Department of Health and Social Security, are as follows:

(1) planning and co-ordinating the provision and development of hospital and specialist services throughout the region, in collaboration with the Boards of Governors of teaching hospitals in the region;

(2) supervising the work of Hospital Management Committees (H.M.C.s) in the region, allocating money and monitoring its use;

(3) appointing members of H.M.C.s and senior medical and dental staff;

(4) planning and executing major building projects within the region;

(5) providing certain direct services, e.g. blood transfusions and mass radiography.

---

[2] The Seebohm Report (1968) foreshadowed the changes made by the Local Authority Social Services Act 1970. Broadly, the basis of the division between health, and social services, functions was according to the expertise required of the providers. Functions which required trained doctors or nurses, for example, were left with health authorities. All the functions that could be carried out by trained social workers in respect of:

(1) children in need,
(2) the mentally disturbed,
(3) the aged,
(4) the sick,
(5) the homeless,

were in general, transferred to the new social services authorities.

It is worth noting that R.H.B.s provide the services of specialists not only within hospitals, but within the clinic or home, if needed – so called 'domiciliary visiting'.

All members of R.H.B.s, including the chairman, are appointed by the Secretary of State, following consultations with professional societies, local authorities, the appropriate university, trade unions, employers' associations and other interested bodies. These bodies may nominate members, but the final decision on appointment clearly rests with the Secretary of State.

The R.H.B. itself appoints a number of chief officers to help carry out its policies, including a Regional Secretary (its senior administrator), a Senior Administrative Medical Officer, a Regional Treasurer, a Regional Architect, a Regional Engineer, a Regional Nursing Officer and so on.

Although the R.H.B. is a body with its own legal existence (so for example, that it can be sued in its own name), it is also described as an agent of the Secretary of State and subject to his regulations and directions.[3]

Hospital Management Committees

Just as R.H.B.s are regional agents of the Secretary of State, so H.M.C.s are local agents of the R.H.B. Again, the H.M.C. has a separate legal identity. Its functions in the words of the 1946 Act are:

'subject to and in accordance with regulations and such directions as may be given by the Minister or the Regional Hospital Board, to control and manage that hospital or group of hospitals on behalf of the Board....' (Section 12)

This involves it in numerous detailed duties such as appointing all hospital staff other than senior medical and dental staff, ensuring the general maintenance of premises and equipment, the purchase of supplies, and so on.

Hospital groups vary widely in size. Some control only one large hospital, often a mental hospital. At the other extreme, a few control as many as twenty hospitals of varying sizes. About one-quarter of all groups in the country are concerned exclusively with

[3] See N.H.S. Act 1946, Section 12.

mental illness, most of the rest being 'general-purpose' groups aiming to provide a wide range of clinical facilities.

All members of H.M.C.s, including Chairmen, are appointed by their R.H.B.s, again following consultation with appropriate local interest-groups. H.M.C.s appoint their own Chief Officers, including a Group Secretary, Group Treasurer, Group Engineer (recently), a Chief or Principal Nursing Officer for the group, etc. The only medical officer at group-level is usually the Chairman of the Group Medical Advisory Committee – a part-time post held by a practising consultant elected by his fellows.

Individual Hospitals

Except where a group consists of one hospital only, no statutorily-defined governing body exists for the individual hospital. In the past it was common for the H.M.C. to appoint a House Committee for each individual hospital – in effect, a sub-committee of the H.M.C. – but House Committees are tending to become more rare following discouragement by various reviewing bodies.[4]

In any case, House Committees could not appoint their own officers. Hospital officers are appointed by the H.M.C., and might include, in a medium or large-size hospital, a Hospital Secretary, a Matron (or more modern equivalent), an Engineer, a Catering Manager, and so on. The range of officers at this level varies considerably with size. A small 'cottage' hospital will have little but nursing staff with a few domestic and clerical helpers. A large district general hospital, the preferred model for the future[5] will have a full range of officers representing all the various occupations found at Group level, and perhaps more. In some cases, particularly those of ex-local-authority hospitals taken into the National Health Service in 1948 (including a large number of mental hospitals), there will be a designated Medical Superintendent[6] for an individual hospital. In most cases however, there will be no full-time appointed medical officer with administrative responsi-

[4] See the Guillebaud Report (1956) paras. 242-248 and the Farquharson-Lang Report (1966) paras. 115-116.

[5] See the Hospital Plan (Ministry of Health 1962) and the Bonham-Carter Report (Department of Health and Social Security (1969)).

[6] The possible variety in content and authority in such a role is discussed in Chapter 5.

bilities in relation to the individual hospital although there will often be a chairman of the medical staff of the hospital, elected by all the consultants who attend the hospital, or by all the general practitioners who form the staff of those hospitals formerly called 'cottage-hospitals', and now more properly named 'general-practitioner hospitals'.

Boards of Governors

The Board of Governors in relation to teaching hospitals combines the role played by R.H.B.s and H.M.C.s in relation to non-teaching hospitals.[7] Each Board is by definition associated with the medical school of a university so that in addition to the provision of normal hospital facilities it must ensure the provision of facilities for clinical teaching and research at either undergraduate or post-graduate level. Each Board carries out its own capital works programme subject to the approval of the Secretary of State. Each has within its purview anything from one to about a dozen individual hospitals.

The Secretary of State appoints the Chairman of the Board and such number of other members as he thinks fit. The universities, the teaching staff of the medical schools, and the associated regional boards each nominate up to one-fifth of the membership. The remainder are appointed after consultation with local health authorities and such other organizations as appear to be concerned.

The Board of Governors again appoints its own officers: a chief administrative officer (known variously as the Secretary, the House Governor, the Administrator, etc.), a Chief Nursing Officer, a Treasurer, an Engineer and so on. As for H.M.C.s, it is unusual for Boards of Governors to appoint a medical officer with full-time administrative duties which span the group.

---

[7] In the last few years a small number of teaching-hospital groups have been established under H.M.C.s within the sphere of R.H.B.s, rather than under Boards of Governors.

Part I
Elements of Hospital Organization

3 The Nature of Organization – An Initial Conception

Organization and Objects

Even when he adopts, as we have done, a client-centred approach, any researcher inevitably brings to the study-situation his own initial conceptions, or (as they are correctly called) his preconceptions. There is of course no need to be apologetic about this fact – the important thing is to be as explicit as possible about these preconceptions in the first place, and then to be prepared to modify them to the extent that they fail, or prove insufficient in testing. Here then, in brief, are our initial conceptions in this project.[1]

First, *organization* implies a group of people working in some structured way towards common ends. (See end of chapter – Note 1.)

The common ends we shall call the *objects* of the organization. (See end of chapter – Note 2.) The structuring of the activities of a particular member so as to contribute to the objects, we shall call an *organizational role*. Each notion requires expansion.

To say that there are common ends is not to imply that each member is, could be, or ought to be, completely in agreement with his fellows as to what is to be done. Each brings his own interests, his own criteria, and his own values; but if there is to be anything recognizable as 'organized' activity, there must be *some* area of consensus, *some* common ground, on what it is all about.

[1] The debt to the work of the Glacier Project (see references to E. Jaques and W. Brown) will be evident. Many of the initial conceptions are common to both projects, though what subsequently emerges shows we believe characteristics and differences particular to the Hospital Service.

It is assumed in this project that individual perceptions about these common objects (like any other perceptions) can be made explicit and compared with each other, and with manifest statements of organizational objects. Differences can be explored, and resolved or exposed. Common ground can be agreed, and used as a basis for further action (including organization-design).

The manifest objects of the present Hospital Service are to be found in legislation. Looking there, we find that the overriding object is 'to promote the establishment in England and Wales of a comprehensive health service designed to secure improvement in the physical and mental health of the people of England and Wales, and the prevention, diagnosis and treatment of illness' and more specifically 'to provide ... hospital accommodation, medical, nursing or other services required at or for the purpose of hospitals ... the services of specialists ... and facilities ... for clinical teaching and research'.[2]

Through individual discussion within the project it is possible to produce more specific statements of objects, and agree them generally with members of the service. More specific statements of objects for the existing Hospital Service are suggested in Chapter 10.

However specific the outcome, the statements will never, of course, exclude the possibility of personal interpretation and value judgements. Just how good a nursing service should be provided? At the expense of *what*? Should more or less emphasis be given to services for the old and mentally-handicapped? Should more comfortable hospital buildings be provided at the expense of more advanced medical equipment? And so on.

Agreement on objects sets firm guide-lines for all activity, but within these guide-lines arguments on more immediate goals, and the priorities to be attached to these, are bound to rage. Indeed, it is just because of this that boards and committees with wide membership are established, to give the broadest possible consideration to alternative policies and priorities, and then to make authoritative judgements on them. Even where costs and benefits may be reduced to the common language of money, many other values resist the translation. Certain major value-judgements will always and inevitably have to be made. The board or committee – like the individual member of the organization – will need some

[2] National Health Service Act, 1946, Sections 1 (1), 3 (1) and 12 (3).

overriding guide for its work, in the form of terms of reference, or of aims and objects as laid down in a binding constitution.

Individual Role

Individual role is the other basic concept of organization. Put another way – people, to the extent they are organized, carry specific and differentiated roles. Commonly, in organizations, these roles are given titles, so that by this they can easily be distinguished from the particular individuals who fill them at particular times. In the Hospital Service titles like 'ward sister' 'hospital engineer' 'group secretary' 'chairman of the medical advisory committee' arise and carry connotations apart from the personal characteristics of *this* particular ward sister or *that* particular hospital engineer.

What are these extra-personal connotations, and how can they be identified and described? (See end of chapter – Note 3.)

Titles only help to the extent that they imply specific functions. Some – 'consultant in neuro-surgery', 'treasurer', 'catering manager' – are rich in associations, and deliver strong indications of role. Others – 'assistant secretary', 'senior nursing officer' – are more neutral. The *minimum* function of a title is simply to distinguish one post from another – theoretically a designating number would do.

The first specification of any role is then, in more or less detail, a statement of the *functions* or *duties* which fall upon any occupant. If one is told that this particular secretary is responsible for planning and progressing building work, or that that particular senior nursing officer is concerned with recruitment and training matters, then the previously unspecific roles begin to come in focus. Such specifications of functions, duties or 'responsibilities' are obviously required from time to time for practical purposes, and are frequently given in greater or lesser detail, for example in many existing types of job-description.

What is less frequently attempted is any specification of the part of any role complementary to its function, that is, the freedom of movement open to the role performer in carrying out his functions, the right of the performer to act at his own discretion; or, the range of *authority*[3] in the role. Can the consultant in neuro-surgery

---

[3] See Newman and Rowbottom (1968, Chapter 2) for a more extended discussion of the nature of organizational authority.

command extended theatre services at his own discretion? Can the treasurer, in his duty of controlling expenditure, veto at his own discretion any items of expenditure by any other officer? Can the catering manager decide for himself whether or not to use regional contracts in buying provisions and food? Can the senior nursing officer in carrying out her training function, direct serving nurses to attend courses as and when she considers it desirable?

Research experience has proved that it is neither possible nor desirable to attempt a systematic specification of all the discretion implicit in any role. However there are usually a few areas in any role where the freedom open to the performer is of critical import-ance and where explicit clarification of limits is helpful both to the performer and others in the situation.

One such area is often authority with regard to cash expenditure. Another – invariably – is any authority in relation to others in the organization, to instruct, to sanction, or both.

Naturally there can be disagreements – open conflicts even – about the duties that particular members ought to carry out, and even more, about their rights in carrying out these duties. It is again part of the research procedure in this particular project to make explicit any such differences in view, with a strong pre-supposition that getting clarity in these matters is often a big step towards resolving them.

The less there is clarity and consensus as to legitimate roles, the more turns on the particular mix of personalities in the situation – with the strongest winning the day. As new group secretaries, or treasurers or medical administrators (or whatever) are appointed, the organization – the actual way decisions get made – changes too in an unpredictable way. Systematic training be-comes impossible if it is not known for what roles people are being trained, and systematic organization change becomes impossible too, since it is impossible to describe either the point of start or the finish.

On the other hand, clarity about individual roles does not preclude freedom of action, nor does it preclude change. It gives the opportunity to be more explicit about what is expected of people as well as the opportunity to give them a defined zone of freedom to act, appropriate to their expectation and to their own abilities (see end of chapter – Note 4). It also gives the chance of controlled organizational change by being able to specify what changes in role are implied by any proposed scheme of change.

Again, when people's freedom to act is made implicit, it can be sanctioned by all concerned. Their interaction with others, their influence on others, can take place in a regularized way, i.e. with authority, in contrast to the precarious route of unregulated personal persuasion and power.

Tasks

It is possible to be more specific about the work to be carried out in a particular role than a mere analysis of continuing duties or functions to be carried out, in whatever detail.

Compare the following sets of statements about the content of roles:

1A The Ward Sister must help in the training of learner nurses allocated to her ward.

1B This particular learner nurse is allocated to this ward for three months. The Ward Sister must ensure that she gets a reasonable amount of practical clinical instruction, and a reasonable variety of exposure to different nursing situations within this time.

2A The Group Engineer must carry out, in addition to ad hoc maintenance, special engineering projects, as authorized.

2B The Group Engineer must ensure that all items on this particular works programme are completed within the year.

3A The Hospital Secretary is responsible for the continual review and development of procedures and systems.

3B The Hospital Secretary must carry out a complete review of the organization of the medical records department and report, with any proposals, within the next six months.

The first statement of each pair is a statement of a continuing duty. The second of each pair poses a specific *objective* to be achieved in a specific period of *time*. This sort of specific description of work we have called a *task*. In each of these pairs of examples, the task quoted in the second statement is a specific manifestation of the more general function described in the first.

In general, it is possible to see the work of anyone as consisting of a continuous series of tasks, some short, some long, and often overlapping. It is arguable that everybody must have in mind some sort of ground-plan of specific targets aimed to be achieved in specific times before they can engage in work, although it is far from the case that people always see their work explicitly in these terms. Some tasks may be explicitly assigned by supervisors ('take this patient to X-ray'); some may be implicit in statements of duties ('after each H.M.C. meeting, produce draft minutes'), many arise at the discretion of the performer, for example, in responding to particular requests for services, or deciding to undertake minor pieces of development work on his own initiative.

Even though the work in any role may be regarded as consisting of a complex of individual tasks, it is not for most practical purposes useful to attempt to specify these comprehensively. Some studies of the task-structure of a number of roles in hospitals are in fact being carried out in this project, with a view to establishing the level of work in the role; but the results are not cleared for general report at the time of writing. (See end of chapter – Note 5.)

Accountability and Sanctions

Once the idea gains acceptance that each person in a hospital (or other organization) has a specific role to play, he becomes not just generally and jointly responsible for all that goes on, but specifically responsible for the way he plays his particular role, well or badly. If he is good at his particular job (whatever it is) enhanced reputation and prospects of promotion may rise for him as an individual, regardless of how the hospital as a whole functions. Or if he is not up to his job he may be transferred or dismissed, again regardless of the quality of work of his colleagues.

This particular and concentrated responsibility of the individual for performance in keeping with the expectation of his own particular role, we have called *accountability*. It implies the presence of a judge somewhere in the situation (exactly where is always a question of great interest, as will become apparent) armed with 'hard' institutionalized sanctions – the right to affect such things as pay, promotion, continued employment or professional membership – as opposed to the 'softer' sanctions of generalized approval or reprobation possessed by all with whom the performer works.

Over and above this the performers will still feel a generalized *sense of responsibility*, in greater or lesser degree for all that hap-

pens within their ken, whether or not it lies within their particular
role to deal with the matters concerned. (In emergencies, all
citizens are firemen, at least until the 'regular' firemen appear.)
In several notorious cases in the hospital world,[4] individual and
junior members of staff have, out of a sense of responsibility,
sounded the alarm about intolerable situations for which they
could not personally be held accountable, whoever else could – and
it is well that they have.

Organization as Role-Structures

The initial conception then, sees hospitals (like other organizations) as groups of people working within a structure of inter-
related roles. Each role is describable in terms of

- (a) the functions or duties to be performed, broken if desired into
  the kinds of task to which they give rise;
- (b) the authority of the occupant, i.e. his right to act at his own
  discretion, within limits;
- (c) the accountability of the occupant for his performance.
  (See end of chapter – Note 6.)

Together, the roles add to a structure whose total effect can be
compared with the overriding objects to be achieved. The prime
test of the efficacy of the total role-structure is whether it does or
not truly and economically achieve the objects, whatever these are
agreed to be. Would a different organization of medical, nursing,
or administrative staff result in better services to patients? A
second test will always be the efficacy with which the role-structure
provides for the needs of the members of the organization – not
only to earn their living, but to express their abilities and concerns, and to develop and progress as individuals. Will (for
example) a particular organization of pharmaceutical staff provide
a satisfactory career-structure, and attract and retain suitable staff?
The two needs will commonly run together but there will
obviously be times when some degree of conflict is involved. At
such points value judgements will then have to be made of just
how much a hospital should bend to the needs of its staff at the
expense of its patients. Ultimately, it has to be accepted that a

4 See the Ely Report (1969) and the Farleigh Report (1971).

hospital is a place for treating patients, not for employing staff in satisfying conditions.[5]

The role-system is as it were, the bone-structure of the organization. The flesh and blood (the particular members of the organization who come and go) may change and be renewed – the bone-structure remains basic and changes only slowly. It provides a stiffening and a durability against this or that transitory shock. Of course, the analogy must not be pressed too far; role-structures, being man-created, can be changed radically and rapidly, should the situation demand it.

Obviously to look at bone-structure is not to look at the whole living, breathing entity. What matters in the end, in hospitals as elsewhere, is what values, attitudes and abilities, individual members bring to bear, how well they communicate and how earnest they are in their desire to co-operate. The study and clarification of roles and role-structure is only justified to the extent that it helps these things; that it may help them decisively is certainly a major premise in this project.

Operational and Other Functions

If the existing role-structure makes any sort of sense, the functions in all the individual roles should, as suggested, in aggregate approximate to the function implicit in the objects – simply, each role should make its particular contribution to the whole enterprise.

However the functions to be carried out in some roles will directly satisfy the specific objects, whilst the functions in other roles will naturally be felt as supportive or secondary. We have called the first *operational functions*, and the roles which include them, *operational roles*. In any pattern of rational organization-design, they must be the first roles to be considered and established. Other 'non-operational' roles, can then be added, as required. (As will become apparent later, it seems that certain characteristic

[5] The inherent tension between the needs of the organization (work-needs, task-needs) on the one hand and the personal needs of the individual member on the other, have been sensitively explored by Argyris in a whole series of works (see for example Argyris, 1964). Jaques' (1967) discussion of the relation between level of work and the different and developing capacities of individual employees is also germane.

types of relationship arise between operational roles, which are different from the types of relationship which arise between non-operational and operational roles.) Thus in hospitals medical and first-level nursing roles, amongst others, are operational because the provision of medical and nursing services is, it is suggested, part of the specific objects of the Hospital Service. On the other hand, the production of accounts, the recruitment of staff, and the provision of supplies, amongst other activities, necessary though they may be, are not in themselves activities which hospitals have been established to pursue. (See end of chapter – Note 7.)

Definition of Concepts

Another major premise of this particular research approach is that the precise definition of the various concepts used in the research is of central importance. Too many otherwise excellent reports[6] on, and studies of, hospital organization have been marred by the use of terms like 'co-ordination', 'management', 'direction', 'co-opera-tion', 'teamwork', 'clinical freedom', 'seniority', 'level', 'grade', etc., in ways which can be interpreted according to individual taste. Naturally, parties with different interests will choose different interpretations. What then happens in subsequent discussion, is that issues of real substance get inextricably mixed in an overlay of semantic confusion.

Another regrettable consequence of the lack of precise descriptive language is that where situations of good organization and good working-relationship have been achieved by chance or by deliberate effort, it is impossible to communicate the beneficial features accurately to others in similar positions. We have frequently been presented in field-work with statements to the effect that, 'the present situation works well' – but what precise organizational arrangement is working well has often proved difficult to elucidate. It need hardly be stressed again that until there is the possibility of precise description of organizational situations – and this requires the existence of significant and defined concepts – there can be no basis for scientific test of organizational alternatives, or systematic dissemination of the alternatives that work best.

[6] The Salmon Report (1966) is an honourable exception here, whether or not one agrees with all its definitions, or finds them uniformly useful. At least one knows exactly what it is with which one is agreeing or disagreeing.

Our attempt throughout the project has been a rigorous definition of all the concepts used and developed. A glossary of the main concepts developed to date is given in Appendix A. We have produced definitions for the basic concepts discussed in this chapter – objects, operational activities, role, duties, authority, accountability. We have produced (tentatively in some cases) definitions of the more specific concepts used in following chapters – superior or managerial roles, service-giving roles, co-ordinating roles, representative roles, hierarchical organization, collegiate organization, committees, etc. It is unlikely that all these definitions will prove 'right'. Modifications will be needed somewhere in the long run; at least it will be clear exactly what it is that is being modified.

Notes to Chapter 3

Note 1. The Definition of Organization (page 25)

The terse definition of organization given above short-cuts a large and important area of discussion amongst sociologists and organization-theorists on what in fact constitutes 'an organization', and what distinguishes it for example, from other social forms and groupings, such as a family, a community, an ethnic group or an occupational group. Many attempted definitions have emphasized just the two features extracted here:

(1) the existence of a definite goal of some kind, or of a number of goals; and

(2) the relative formality of social relationships amongst those within the organization.

(Silverman, 1970 page 9, provides a useful summary of various views and definitions.)

How are the goals defined, and who defines them? Clearly, the private goals, or 'motives' of organization-members, must be distinguished from goals with some more public status (Gross 1969). But after this the real uncertainty arises. One school of thought, the 'systems' school (for example Katz and Kahn 1966, Miller and Rice 1967) tends to see organizational goals as immanent in the function of the organization in its larger society. Miller and Rice (1967) talk of the 'primary task' which must be inferred from how the organization actually behaves or functions in its environment (page 27). (Silverman's criticism of this procedure from an 'action' framework is no doubt accurate.) Perrow (1970, page 134) draws attention to the fact that different groups associated with an organization, the manager, the customer, society at large, may be expected to have different and conflicting definitions of goal.

This leads to a second view that the study of organizational goals must proceed from consideration of statements from the various actors in the situation. Etzioni (1964) in effect proposes this approach, but for safety, as one might say, combines it with direct observation and inference as well, in an attempt to establish the 'real' goals (page 7). He emphasizes the well-established phenomenon of 'displacement' – the tendency for the behaviour of members of organizations to shift from originally-stated ends to necessary means as a primary orientation.

In this research the emphasis is solely and unequivocally on *statement* as a source of knowledge of organizational goals; and the difference between original statements and the working supposition of the many actors in the situation is analysed in terms of concepts of *manifest, assumed* and *extant situations* within the framework of a planned-change process which moves always to a consensus of agreement on statements of the *requisite* (see Appendix B). Displacement, in other words is regarded as evidence of some social-pathology.

As far as formality of social relationships is concerned, it is evident that so far as they are consciously created organizations may well be expected to exhibit bureaucratic characteristics in the Weberian sense; for example, the existence of explicit rules and administrative regulations, methodical provision for the allocation of duties, appointment on the basis of personal ability, a hierarchy of authority and so on. More generally, the internal structure of organizations across many cultures will depend on the 'social technology available at the time' as Stinchcombe (1969, page 153) has pointed out, and may lack full characteristics of bureaucracy in primitive societies, or for example 'family' firms.

Note 2. 'Objects and Goals' (page 25)

The word 'objects' rather than the more general term 'goals' has been used just to emphasize the institutionalized, man-made, and consensual nature of organizational-goals. After all, such goals may have (and often do have) existence on paper, in statements of legislation, 'aims and objects' clauses of written constitutions, etc., whose social status is far beyond that of an idle observation or description. Nor need the fact that such statements represent, or strive to represent, a consensus view at any time, obscure the fact that there may well have been conflicts of opinion prior to their formulation and agreement, and that there may well be conflicts at any time thereafter as to their continuing appropriateness. To assert that there is such a thing as social structure is not to affirm that it has been readily created, or that it is immune to the pressures of change.

Note 3. The Description of Role (page 27)

This of course is the classical field of role-theory. As stated here the question deliberately assumes an approach to role in terms of given and external expectations rather than in terms of the voluntary assumption of sets of behaviour by the actor; that is, the approach is broadly sociological (at least, in its more structural interpretation) rather than psychological or dramaturgical (Biddle and Thomas, 1966, page 13).

Immediately, of course, the question arises, whose expectations define the role where conflicting expectations exist. Gross et al (1957) point out that role-conflict can mean (amongst other things) both difference in view of the actor's role held by a number of people in the situation which may or may not be perceived by the actor, and difference in perception reported by the actor himself. Again the question arises whether the content of roles can most properly be established by observation of behaviour, or by collection of explicit statements (Nadel 1957, page 25). This research clearly rests on the use of explicit statement rather than direct observation of behaviour (see Appendix B). Some degree of role-conflict is assumed to be the normal starting point in a situation presenting organizational problems. The doubt may either be in the mind of one actor or in the minds of the many actors in the 'role-set', or both. The point of the project-method is to make these doubts explicit with a view to establishing consensus on what statement of role is *requisite*.

Note 4. Freedom within Role (page 28)

The problem of the varying ways in which roles are performed by different performers has been a constant headache to the role-theorist. Does it mean that all real-life performances exhibit some or other degree of (reprehensible) deviance from the one ideal role-performance? Or does it indicate a total lack of consensus on what constitutes the ideal role-performance? Surely the more useful view is that roles can be specified in such a way as to give individual performers freedom to interpret them as they think best, provided that they stay within certain agreed limits. Beyond these, lies genuine 'deviance'. Within this lies genuine freedom of personal expression.

This view is in line with Nadel's (1957) observation that the rules of role-behaviour, like those of a game, whilst disallowing certain options do allow many options and a degree of latitude (page 41). It also fits with Jackson's (1966) presentations of a norm as applying to a *range* of tolerable behaviours, rather than one specific behaviour.

Note 5. The Analysis of the Task-Content of Roles (page 30)

One reason for task-analysis is as a necessary prerequisite to measuring 'level of work' as defined by Jaques (1956, 1967). Jaques' theory of measurement of level of work (or responsibility) is based on 'time-span of discretion' which is defined (broadly) in terms of the longest (sanctioned) task in a role. Jaques (op. cit) reported relationships between level of work (measured in this way) and the 'felt-fair pay' feeling expressed by the role-holders. Richardson (1971) confirmed these findings. Jaques' consequent theory of the relationship between levels of work and the optimum number of management levels in hierarchical organization is expounded in *Glacier Project Papers* (Brown and Jaques 1965). If valid, this has highly important implications for the optimum number of management levels in hospitals of various sizes.

Another, and perhaps more general motive for studying work in task-terms is of course apparent whenever 'management-by-objective' schemes are under trial. Although 'key-results' required, and 'performance standards' (to use the terminology of Humble 1970) do not necessarily themselves constitute specific tasks, it is stressed that explicit time-targets for reaching certain standards or improvements in standard should be set whenever possible.

Note 6. The Basic Content of Organizational Role-Description (page 31)

The basic terms of role-description being established in this particular context then, are those of *title, function* (or *duty*), and *authority*. In addition *accountability* is noted as a feature of all organizational-roles. As Biddle and Thomas (1966, page 8) have convincingly demonstrated there is at present no general consensus on the meanings to be ascribed to various terms in common use in this field – 'position', 'norm', 'sanction', 'status' or even 'role' itself. Nevertheless, in order to emphasize the relationship of the analysis here to role-theory more generally it may be noted that

(a) 'title' is roughly equivalent to *position* in the social structure,
(b) 'duty' or 'function' denotes broadly the positive *obligations* binding on the incumbent,
(c) 'authority' denotes broadly the *rights* of the incumbent, what he may legitimately expect by way of compliance from others.

Note 7. The Nature of Operational and Non-Operational Work (page 33)

We are still struggling with the exact categorization of work into its various operational and non-operational kinds – and indeed with the problem of finding a more adequate and flattering alternative to 'non-operational' as a title! The earlier Glacier categories for instance, of *development, manufacturing,* and *selling,* for operational work, and of *programming, personnel* and *technical* for 'non-operational' or 'specialist' work (Brown 1960) have not proved easily applicable, even with obvious translation, to hospital work.

A possible, but as yet highly tentative alternative classification, might be as follows:

operational work
    (1) research into characteristics of the operational field, and evaluation of existing operational services;
    (2) planning and development of new operational services;
    (3) delivery of operational services;

other (non-operational) work
    (1) provision of (trained) personnel;
    (2) provision of other supporting services and resources (logistics);
    (3) managerial, co-ordinating and other inter-role activities of various kinds (e.g. induction, task-setting, monitoring, appraisal etc.);
    (4) financial work;
    (5) secretarial and legal work;
    (6) public relations and fund-raising work.

(See fuller discussion of this point in Chapter 13.)

In systems-theory language, operational activities are those that directly culminate in the outputs of the organization as a whole. The distinction between operational and non-operational activities as defined here is very similar, for example, to the distinction drawn by Miller and Rice (1967) between *operating* activities on the one hand and *maintenance* and *regulating* activities on the other. (Chapter 1.)

'Operating activities (are those) ... that directly contribute to the upkeep, conversion and export processes which define the nature of the enterprise or unit and differentiate it from other enterprises or units ...

Maintenance activities procure and replenish the resources that produce operating activities ...

Regulating activities relate operating activities to each other, maintenance activities to operating activities, and all internal activities of the enterprise (or unit) to its environment.'

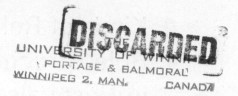

4 Kinds of Roles and Role-Structures in Hospitals

In this chapter research findings on the various kinds of roles and role-structure that have been discovered in the hospital situation will be presented. The other basic organizational feature – the nature of the detailed objects of the Hospital Service will be left till later.

A number of definitions will be quoted. It must be emphasized at the outset that these definitions have not been imported ready-made into the situation, to be applied in any procrustean way. Certain starting definitions were, it is true, brought in from the Glacier Project,[1] but most if not all of these have had to be modified or generalized so as to fit both industrial and social service organization, and many new and important definitions have had to be created. The creation and testing of appropriate ways of describing hospital organization has indeed been a major part of the research work to date, and what is presented is, in an important way, research data in itself.[2]

The way in which organizational roles may be described in terms of functions, authority, and accountability, has been discussed in

[1] See for example, Brown (1960) *Exploration in Management.*

[2] The definitions given in Appendix A represent (with some minor amendments) a list evolved by field-work. After discussion in some dozens of research conferences with senior officers of the N.W. Metropolitan Region, they have been approved and formally adopted by the N.W. Metropolitan Board itself, in June 1971, for the purposes of organizational description, development and specification. As will be described in Appendix B, one of the unusual features of this particular research-approach (social analysis) is that its prime research data arises in the form of *agreed statements*, rather than in the form of independent observation by the researchers.

the last chapter. In our project-work to date, many hundreds of different roles in the Hospital Service have been analysed in this way, and it has become possible to see a number of broad categories of similarity.[3]

One obvious similarity is in work carried out in relation to the Service as a whole. Categories here – nursing, catering, engineering, physiotherapy, etc., are straightforward enough and need no further discussion.

Another way of classifying roles, which cuts across all these conventional categories, is in terms of the kinds of relationships they bear to one another. Appropriate categories here, to illustrate the sort of thing in mind, have names like, 'managerial', 'treatment-prescribing', 'representative', and 'co-ordinating'. They all imply qualities of relationship with other roles: of functions in relation to other roles, authority in relation to the occupants of other roles, and accountability to the occupants of other roles. They speak, then, of the internal structure of the role-system, rather than its function as a whole.

Again the point must be emphasized about the way in which the definition of these various categories has been reached. It has not been our object in this research to attempt to describe and categorize role relationships merely according to the various features that immediately and straightforwardly present themselves in a variety of actual situations – a sort of 'natural-history' approach. On the contrary, in the common absence of clarity about who is accountable to whom, and who has authority to instruct whom on this or that issue, there is no 'straightforward' situation to be described. This study is essentially a process of clarification, starting with such piecemeal statements and assumptions of relationship and function as immediately exist, but aimed from the start at reaching agreements as to what is *requisite*. On occasion, of course, the pre-existing situation may be clear and explicit enough, whether or not it is requisite. Thus, in the terms used in this research, it is possible to distinguish the *extant* situation from what might well be a different *requisite* situation.

Requisite by what test though? As a short answer: requisite in the eyes of all those involved in the analysis at any particular stage, given their perceptions of the work to be done on the one hand, and the resources available to do it on the other. More generally, the search for requisite organization implies consideration of the tasks to be carried out, of the technologies and programmes employed, of the environment to be worked in, and of the characteristics of the people and other resources available. 'Requisite', then, certainly involves consideration amongst other things of the needs, responses and abilities of the human actors in the situation, and where by definition the concern is with establishing requisite modes of interrelationships between roles, these factors become paramount (See end of chapter – Note 1.)

Superior-Subordinate (or Managerial) Relationships

The approach can best be illustrated by taking a specific example from the project. One of the first role relationships that we attempted to get in perspective was that between any person broadly describable as a head, chief, or 'boss', and any one of his or her immediate assistants. Was there in essence (that is, requisitely) a similar relationship to be discerned:

- between the matron of a small hospital and one of her nursing sisters;
- between a consultant and his registrar;
- between a hospital secretary and one of his senior clerical staff;
- between a catering manager and his kitchen superintendent?

Would such a standardized relationship suitably cover the relationship of:

- the group secretary to all other senior officers of the H.M.C.;
- any nurse in one 'Salmon' grade to any other associated nurse in the next lower grade;
- the registrar to the houseman;
- the consultant to the ward sister;
- to take more extreme cases, the R.H.B. as a body, to the H.M.C., as a body?

The difficulty was in seeing which of these relationships were essentially the same, and which were different in some significant[4]

---

[4] Of course, all turns on what differences are 'significant'. The judgement of the researcher is inevitable here; but in the ultimate the check is whether or not any proposed distinction is felt by those with whom we work in the hospital service, to be useful.

degree. (As it turns out, the answer to the first set of questions was probably yes: the answer to the second was probably no – at least in most situations.) We set as a firm research principle that when we came across significant differences in relationships we would not attempt to subsume the various cases into one category, under one title, but would assume that another category and name was going to be necessary. Put another way, none of our definitions of relationship would contain optional or alternative elements, each would cover one unique case.

It certainly was not the case that all people in the first category immediately perceived their inter-relationships in the same terms. The point was that most in that particular list, *following discussion and analysis*, agreed similar sets of characteristics as requisite in their situation. These sets of characteristics were seen as in keeping with normal human expectations and responses in their particular situations and as exhibiting internal consistency.

In a *superior-subordinate (or managerial)* relationship, where a superior A is accountable for ensuring that certain work is carried out and has a subordinate B to assist him in this work, it is requisite that:

(1) A may prescribe B's work and assign tasks to him;
(2) A may veto the appointment of B to the role;
(3) A may apply sanctions to B (the chief sanction in the Hospital Service being the recording of assessments of performance in such a way as to affect B's future career);
(4) A may initiate the transfer of B from the particular role he carries, where he judges his performance not to reach an adequate standard.[5]

[5] We used as a starting point for explorations here the definition of the managerial role that had been evolved in the Glacier Project.

'*Managerial Role.* A role which has subordinate to it, authorized roles; the work of these subordinate roles is determined by the occupant of the managerial role (the manager). The manager is accountable for his subordinate's work and minimally has authority to appoint employees to the subordinate role, to remove them from these roles, and to determine, within whatever policies he is set by higher authority, the differential rewards of his subordinates.' (Brown and Jaques, 1965, page 17.)

The right of a superior to affect the monetary rewards of his subordinates is not generally seen as a realistic (or desirable) sanction by most people with whom we have discussed the matter in the Hospital Service. It is accordingly omitted from the definition. Whether it is requisite at some deeper level is another matter.

In discussion of this definition the logic has usually proved persuasive, that, if A is to be held accountable for the work of B it is requisite that he possess all the elements of authority listed in (1) to (4) above. For if A lacks any of them in a situation where he is being taken to task for shortcomings in the work of his subordinates he can always retort: 'how can I be held accountable for people over whose work I have no control, or in respect of whom I have no sanction, or whom I consider unsuited for the job?' Even then, in a sense he may still be held accountable, but his manifest lack of authority will always buffer him against personal blame for the shortcomings of his so-called subordinates when brought to the test.

On the other hand, it is evidently far from the case that all members of the Hospital Service who consider themselves, or might be considered by others, to approximate to this managerial position do clearly and explicitly carry this full degree of authority. Many in such situations find themselves excluded from appointment panels; often the mechanism for the formal assessment of subordinates is absent, or inappropriate; often, any mechanism for securing the transfer or dismissal of unsatisfactory subordinates is remote and ineffectual. The point is, once again, that there can be general agreement that such a package of role-properties is requisite in situations where a high degree of managerial accountability and control is required, and that such a set of properties may then be used as a standard against which a large range of real-life variants of more or less similarity may be compared.

The characteristics described above are the bare structural bones of the superior-subordinate relationship. Project-work has in fact established a more extended list of the requisite functions of the superior in respect of his subordinates:

(1) participating in selection;
(2) carrying out, or arranging for, induction;
(3) explaining duties, and assigning particular tasks; prescribing methods and programmes of work; assigning resources;
(4) helping with work problems, or with personal problems bearing on work; negotiating personal working-arrangements (leave, duty, etc.);
(5) reviewing performance and general conformity to policy and custom;
(6) assessing suitability for present work, for extended or reduced role, for promotion;

(7) providing or arranging training;

(8) (in extreme cases) initiating transfer or dismissal.

As will be shown, the superior may get help in carrying out these managerial functions in several different ways; but his final decision on the ability of his subordinate, on the latter's suitability for the role, and on the appropriate kind and level of work for him within the role, the superior cannot delegate: they are essential and definite functions. The way in which a superior carries out these functions, the style he employs – authoritarian, neutral, supportive, permissive, participative, etc. is another matter and clearly one of importance but it has not come within the scope of this research. (See end of chapter – Note 2.)

The Treatment-Prescribing Relationship

Having defined in the research an exact point of reference in the superior-subordinate relationship, it then rapidly became apparent that we needed to distinguish a number of other types of relationships which exhibited similarities at first sight.

First we noted that the relationships of doctors to nurses did not (or not generally) wholly fit the superior-subordinate pattern, nor was such seen as desirable. The surface similarity here was that doctors could prescribe the work – indeed the tasks – of nurses. On the other hand they were clearly not regarded, nor regarded themselves, as accountable for the provision of nursing services. The definition which emerged from discussion as requisite to meet the common needs of this situation, ran as follows.

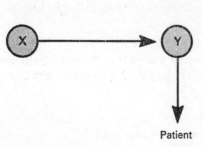

Patient

(1) A treatment-prescribing relationship arises where X (a doctor, say) has authority to prescribe the treatment that Y must give to a patient, or the specific services that are required to be carried out in the course of furthering individual treatments.

(2) X must deal with queries on treatment or services posed by Y, and monitor the treatments and services actually given.

Y might carry out the prescribed treatment-tasks or services himself (or herself), or might delegate them to his (or her) subordinates – for example in the case of a ward sister. Either way, Y would be accountable to his (or her) own superior for observing the treatment-prescriptions and for the way in which they were put into practice.

Supervisory Relationship

At a later stage we distinguished again from the superior-subordinate relationship what (borrowing a term from the Glacier Project[6]) could be called a *supervisory* relationship. It became obvious for example that nurses in many situations, though playing a controlling or directive role in relation to more junior grades, were not (and properly not requisitely) carrying the full range of managerial functions. This was often the case for staff nurses, sometimes for charge nurses in particular situations, and sometimes for nursing officer and even senior nursing officer grades. The nurse concerned would help in dealing with work problems and give instructions and guidance, but in spite of this it would be observable that there was a strong organizational link between her own superior and the nurses she herself supervised. Was this bypassing simply an indication that the superior concerned had not learned to delegate? Or was it that the superior and others had accepted an organizational reality for which the official statements on organization had not allowed?

Again, the situation of the registrar in relation to the houseman could not quite be described as managerial. The houseman certainly looked to the registrar for guidance and instruction on many occasions, but it was the consultant whom he unhesitatingly identified as his 'boss'.

Gradually we established a new role specification.

A supervisory relationship arises where a superior A needs help in managing the work of his subordinates B, in all its aspects. Specifically, the supervisor will help A:
   (1) to induct B into his duties;
   (2) to assign work to B;
   (3) to deal with the immediate work-problems of B;
   (4) to monitor the performance of B;
   (5) to assess the performance of B.

   [6] See Brown 1960, Chapter 14.

The supervisor will have authority to prescribe B's work, but will not have the right of veto on the appointment of B, the right to apply sanctions to B, or to initiate his transfer (or dismissal). These are the definitive rights of the superior which he cannot delegate to the supervisor. Lacking this authority the supervisor cannot be said to be accountable for the work of those he supervises (without further qualification) in the way that the superior is. It is perhaps easier to think of the supervisor as simply being accountable for 'carrying out adequate processes of supervision'.[7]

Co-ordinating Relationship

Awareness of a fourth kind of controlling relationship arose in the first place out of discussion and analysis of the typical role of the Group Secretary. The specific statement that emerged we called a co-ordinating relationship. It gave us great difficulty in precise formulation, and even now may need further refinement or elaboration of definition. It was not (as far as can be discovered) a role for which precise formulation has been attempted hitherto, but it is probably a role of decisive importance in any future organization of the service. (See Chapter 12.)

The problem was this. A number of Group Secretaries with whom we had discussions, whilst they saw certain officers in straightforward subordinate relation to them, saw a number of others (the exact composition of the list varied from place to place, but included such people as the Chief Nursing Officer, the Treasurer, and the Group Engineer) as something less than equal colleagues, but as something more than subordinates. The classic phrase 'first among equals' was regularly paraded to describe this situation.[8]

---

[7] It might be argued by the same token that the superior was simply accountable for 'carrying out adequate processes of management'. Both superior and supervisor carry accountability in some degree for the work of others. The crucial difference is in the degree of authority they possess, which of course, affects what happens in situations where they are being 'brought to account'.

[8] The Bradbeer Report (1954) had of course spoken of the special co-ordinating role of the chief administrator in respect of his colleagues in 'tripartite management', but a precise definition of the co-ordinating role was not attempted in that Report.

Our first attempts at definition in the situation we christened a 'monitoring and co-ordinating' (as opposed to a simple 'co-ordinating') relationship. It included at that time such functions (amongst others) as: monitoring all activities of those subject to the relationship, on behalf of the employing authority; induction; and some element of personal assessment or appraisal. Later we came to see that there were a number of confusions rampant in this first definition. Firstly, we were mixing the specific role of the Group Secretary (see Chapter 9) with a more general definition of a co-ordinating role, which might apply to officers and employees in many other positions. Secondly we were confusing two separate roles, the co-ordinating role and the monitoring role (see below), which really required separate definition. Out latest definition of the co-ordinating role now reads as follows:

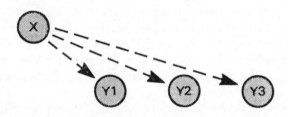

1. *A co-ordinating role* arises where it is felt necessary to establish one person, with the function of co-ordinating the work of a number of others in certain respects, and where a managerial, supervisory or staff relationship is inappropriate. The activity to be co-ordinated might for example be:
   – the production of a report, estimate, plan, or proposal on policy;
   – the implementation of an approved scheme or project;
   – the overcoming of some unforeseen problem affecting normal work.
2. In all cases the co-ordinator can only work within the framework of some specific *task* whose definition is agreeable to all concerned.
3. Specifically, X in a co-ordinating role is accountable in relation to the task concerned for:
   3.1 negotiating co-ordinated work programmes;
   3.2 arranging the allocation of existing resources or seeking additional resources where necessary;
   3.3 monitoring (q.v.) actual progress;

3.4 helping to overcome problems encountered by Y₁, Y₂, etc.

3.5 reporting on progress to those who established the co-ordinating role.

4. In carrying out these activities the co-ordinator X has authority to make firm proposals for action, to arrange meetings, to obtain first-hand knowledge of progress, etc., and to decide what shall be done in situations of uncertainty, but he has no authority in case of sustained disagreements to issue overriding instructions. Y₁, Y₂, etc., have always the right of direct access to the higher authorities who are setting or sanctioning the tasks to be co-ordinated.

5. It is not part of the co-ordinator's role to make formal assessments of the general quality of the performance of those he co-ordinates.

6. There may be situations in which a co-ordinating role is played by a small group, e.g. a committee, rather than by an individual.

Further implications of this definition (like others presented at this point) are discussed in later chapters.

Monitoring Relationship

As we evolved from the notion of one combined monitoring and co-ordinating relationship, it was relatively easy to recognize some specialized roles in hospitals which consisted simply of a monitoring *without* a co-ordinating element. The roles of such people as designated control-of-infections officer in a hospital (usually a consultant pathologist) in relation to sources of potential cross-infection, pharmacist in relation to the control and recording of use of drugs, and designated fire-officer (often the group engineer) in relation to fire risks, for example, conformed to a single type which could be defined as follows.

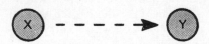

1. *A monitoring role* X arises where it is felt necessary to ensure that the activities of Y conform to adequate standards in some particular respect, and where a managerial, supervisory, or staff, relationship is impossible or needs supplementing. The field of performance being monitored might for example be:
   – adherence to the letter of contract of employment (attendance, hours of work for example);

- adherence to the substance of contract of employment (quantity or quality of work produced);
- adherence to regulations;
- safety;
- financial propriety;
- level of expenditure;
- technical standard of work;
- progress on specific project.

2. Two broad categories of monitoring will be:
  2.1 monitoring in respect of adherence to limiting conditions (minimum standards, regulations, etc.);
  2.2 monitoring in respect of standards achieved within limiting conditions.

  Any given monitoring role may be concerned with the first only, or with both.

3. Specifically, X in a monitoring role is accountable for:
  3.1 ensuring that he is adequately informed of the effects of Y's performance in the field concerned;
  3.2 negotiating improvements with Y where necessary, or failing satisfaction, with Y's superiors;
  3.3 reporting to the higher authorities to whom he is accountable sustained or significant departures in the field concerned;
  3.4 recommending definitions of standards or changes to standards where required.

4. The monitor X has authority:
  4.1 to obtain first-hand knowledge of Y's activities and problems concerning adherence to the limiting requirements;
  4.2 to persuade Y to modify his performance, but not to instruct him.

5. The monitoring role is often combined with an advisory role where special expertise is involved in the monitoring function.

6. It is not part of the role of the monitor to make formal assessments of the general quality of Y's performance – this is the prerogative of the managerial role, if such exists.

7. It is possible that roles exist which carry out some but not all of full-monitoring functions. A *scanning* role for example might be established in order to provide information about actual performance in the field concerned, without having also the function of evaluating deviations or of negotiating improvements.

8. There may be situations in which a monitoring role is played in full or part by a small group of people, e.g. a committee, rather than by an individual.

The Relationships of Boards and Committees to their Chief Officers, Agents and Appointees

A considerable area of doubt exists at the time of writing about the exact quality of requisite relationships of boards (R.H.B.s, H.M.C.s, etc.) to their chief officers, agents and other appointees. Are these all, essentially superior-subordinate relationships as defined above? Several arguments suggest not. For one thing, the superior-subordinate relationship is most easily conceived as existing between two individuals. Where the higher party is a composite body, the whole social atmosphere just *feels* different. It is not for example immediately easy to conceive of any chief officer of a hospital authority as an *assistant* to some principal (he is in a sense, the principal). It becomes even more difficult to entertain the idea of a straightforward superior-subordinate relationship where *both* parties to the relationship are composite bodies; for example, as might be the situation between the present R.H.B. and H.M.C. or between the Regional Health Authority and Area Health Authority planned for the reorganized service.

The most persuasive argument for an essential difference arises, however, in connection with the idea of *task* (see Chapter 3). A governing body, as an entity, cannot by its composite and occasional nature carry out substantive tasks, beyond its own tasks of deliberation at meetings. Substantive tasks to promote the objects of the organization have perforce to be carried out by executive officers or by individual members of the governing body acting in an executive capacity. The governing body of the organization can *sanction* the tasks being performed by officers, and it can *initiate* them. It can set *policy* in regard to them and pass *judgements* upon them. But it cannot, in a substantial sense, *participate* in these tasks. In the end, if an individual officer is incapable of carrying out his tasks, the governing body cannot perform them for him, or even help him perform them, they can only look for another officer.

But a real superior *can* help his subordinate to carry out tasks, if needs be. He can withdraw work back to himself if the work he has delegated to his subordinate becomes too onerous. The cycle of – assessment – delegation of work – reassessment – adjustment of work, is characteristic of the managerial role, and arguably does not occur in quite the same way in the relation of board to officer, or board to subordinate board.

There is probably a further distinction still to be made between those who are felt to be (and referred to) as the 'officers' of a governing body – its secretary, its treasurer, etc., and those like medical consultants, who are not in the same way the executors of its instructions and policy.

In short, there are probably further significant variants of controlling or directing relationships yet to be defined, to cover the position of a governing body in relation to its officers, to its subsidiary governing bodies, and to its employed professional practitioners.[9]

Collateral, Service and Similar Colleague-Type Relationships

So far, the relationships discussed have all been of the 'up-and-down' variety; what about the 'sideways' relationships?[10]

The most straightforward discovered and identified in the research were those between certain pairs of colleagues where both members of the pair were carrying out operational work, where the work of both interacted, and where both were subject to the authority of some common superior, immediately or at some point organizationally-removed.

For example, C2 and C3 (see Figure 4.1) might be a clinical instructor, and a ward sister, respectively. Now (as will be argued in Chapter 10) both nurse-training and service-nursing are operational activities of the Hospital Service, with the implication that neither has precedence over the other. The clinical instructor cannot have final precedence over the ward sister (or vice versa) because nurse-training does not have final preference over service-nursing (or vice versa). Where arrangements for the training of particular nurses are concerned, mutual agreement has to be

[9] We are currently considering the possibility of changing 'superior-subordinate' to 'manager-subordinate', thus releasing the former expression for the general name of a whole class of relations where one person or body has authority of some kind in respect of another, and reserving the second for the specific cluster of functions and authority which may arise between two individuals, as defined above.

[10] Such relationships are rarely taken as a usual feature of so-called 'bureaucratic' organization. All too often they are dismissed as mere 'informal' organization. It is our view however that such relationships are just as capable of 'formulation', i.e. of explicit and agreed definition, as the 'vertical' relationships to which overwhelming attention is paid.

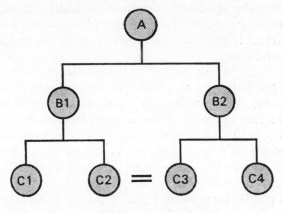

Figure 4.1

reached by ward and teaching staff, taking each situation on its own merits. If significant disagreements arise on specific occasions, or a succession of disagreements betokening some long-standing problem, then the two nurses concerned have to refer them to their immediate superiors for guidance. If these cannot resolve the matter satisfactorily, the matter must be referred to the next level, and so on, until a *cross-over point* (Role A in Figure 4.1) is reached. In this example, the cross-over point would be the Chief Nursing Officer of the Hospital Group. He or she would have authority to resolve the matter in a particular case, or to set new policies where a long standing problem arose. We have called such, collateral relationships.

(1) A *collateral* relationship arises where the work of two people, ultimately subject to the authority of a common superior, interacts in such a way that mutual accommodation is needed in certain decisions, and where neither has authority over the other.

(2) Where collateral colleagues disagree ultimate resolution can be found at the cross-over point represented by that common superior.

Straightforward collateral relationships in hospitals, as defined thus, are not as common as might be supposed at first, since not only do they imply significant interacting decisions, but also the presence of one unequivocal hierarchy of full superior-subordinate relationships, culminating in a cross-over point. As will be suggested later, the apparent reality of typical hospital organization is not that of one monolithic hierarchy, but rather of a large number of separate hierarchies, each subject only to the authority of the governing body.

May this governing body be thought of as a cross-over point? Where it has authority to adjudicate on disputed issues, perhaps it usefully may; and therefore the relationship between members of separate hierarchies as far as these issues are concerned, is collateral. The danger is in assuming that the governing body will be a cross-over point for all disputed issues, as in fact it may lack recognized authority on the issue concerned. For example, if a consultant surgeon and a consultant paediatrician disagree about the treatment of a particular patient, their 'superior' body (the R.H.B., say) cannot appropriately adjudicate – it must be left to other mechanisms, such as professional etiquette on who had prime care of the patient.

In fact, there are a variety of types of relationships between interacting colleagues in the hospital situation from collateral in the sense defined above (that is within one all-embracing hierarchy) to those at the other extreme effectively quite without a 'cross-over point', like relationships between fellow-consultants, or relationships between consultants and general practitioners, or between consultants and local authority social workers, for example. Again, these further varieties of colleague-relationships still require precise identification and definition at this stage of the research.

There is however, another variety of 'sideways' relationship which is quite obviously different from collateral, and which has in fact been distinguished and precisely identified. This is the 'service-giving' relationship. In none of the examples mentioned above can it be said that one party is there to serve the other. Clinical instructors are not there to serve ward sisters, or vice versa. Paediatricians are not there to serve surgeons. Surgeons are not there to serve general practitioners, or social workers. On the other hand medical secretarial staff are in being to serve doctors, and staff of nurses' residences to serve nurses. The chief *raison d'être* of many categories of staff in hospitals – supplies officers, engineers, typists, laundry staff – is not themselves directly to provide services to patients, but to provide services to those who do serve patients or to those who carry out other kinds of operational work. Service-providers are essentially resource-providers. The quality of their resources, of their work, may very well bear on the patient; but interposed, as it were, between the resource-provider and the patient are other staff with operational roles who have the duty of checking the quality of these resources before they become transformed in services to patients.

In a general sense then, all providers of resources are service-givers, as opposed to operational-role performers. However, we have in this project-work restricted the term 'service-giving' to a more specific situation where:

(a) the service-seeker may decide what services they require at their own discretion (within certain limits) occasion by occasion – as opposed to the situation where the services to be provided have already been specified and programmed elsewhere;

(b) both service-users and service-givers are subject to one common, 'cross-over point' superior.

With these conditions in mind the following definition has been evolved.

A service relationship is one where:

(1) one or more people may request at their discretion certain services from the person in the service-giving role, within certain limits on kinds of service to be made available;

(2) the service-giver is accountable for providing such services, within the limits of his own resources and policies on the kinds of service available;

(3) the common superior at the cross-over point can receive any unresolved questions of quality or priority of service, and can set common policies within which both service-seekers and service-givers must operate.

Now just as a collateral relationship represents the most fully-structured example of a whole family of colleague-relationships, whose other members are less fully-structured in varying degrees, so the same applies in service-giving. None of the following situations quite accords with service-giving as defined above, though all can be argued in one sense or other to be service-type situations in a more general sense.

– Medical secretaries, in relationships to hospital doctors. The group secretary may set binding policies as far as secretaries are concerned, but neither he, nor the H.M.C., nor the R.H.B., can set

policies which are binding on the doctors – they can merely offer
to extend or contract the services available.
- Engineers and builders in relation to ward nursing staff, as far
as new facilities or major alterations are concerned. Ward nursing
staff cannot requisition new facilities or major alterations at their
own discretion, though they may requisition maintenance work
on existing physical facilities.
- Pathologists in relation to surgeons or physicians. There is no
cross-over superior who can set binding policies for both parties.
Pathologists must themselves judge where requests for investigations are beyond the bounds of what is necessary or practicable,
or of what is established within the meaning of 'pathology-work'
at any given point of medical evolution.

(Again, as in the case of collateral relationships, a further series
of relationships like service-giving, but with some significant variations, awaits more precise identification and definition.)

Deputies, Assistants, and Staff Officers

An early problem in the research arose in connection with analysing the roles of deputies and assistants. Such titles are in frequent
use in certain parts of the Service.[11] What is the exact content of
the role, in each case? There are really two separate questions to
be asked of anybody designated deputy – what does he do when
the boss is there, and what does he do when he is away?

The second is much easier to answer. The answer, in general
terms, is that the deputy, in the absence of his superior, makes
such decisions as he has to, taking due account of the likely period
of absence of the superior. He takes on part of the role of his
superior, but just how much depends on the particular situation.
In other words, if the boss is away for an hour, little more than
fire-alarms and other extreme urgencies require the deputy's attention. If he is away for several days, urgent correspondence and
other urgent operational problems may need attendance. If he is
away for several months, whole systems of work may need adjustment, or discussion on staff replacements may be needed.

This measured stepping into the superior's role is the activity of

[11] The use of 'deputy' and 'assistant' in nursing, as in 'assistant matron',
has fallen-out of favour following Salmon's strictures (1966 para. 3.37). Will
these titles rise again? See Chapter 7.

deputizing.[12] Seen as an occasional activity, and not as a full-time role in itself, it is evident that it can be assigned to any one of the superior's existing subordinates and does not necessarily require the setting-up of a full-time additional role.

In order to assess what a so-called full-time deputy might do in the *presence* of his boss, it is necessary, first to consider another organizational concept, that of 'staff officer'. In hospital project-work, one of the concepts with which we started out was that of staff officer as it had been elaborated and defined in the Glacier Project.[13]

In the Glacier Metal Company, a manufacturing concern, three kinds of roles were identified which had accountability for the planning or support of manufacturing operations, rather than for the operations themselves. These were:

(a) *personnel-officer roles* – concerned with recruitment, welfare, training, payment systems, and other general organizational and personnel matters;

(b) *production engineering roles* – concerned with manufacturing methods, equipment, and standards of manufacture;

(c) *production control or programming roles* – concerned with planning and co-ordinating the balance, quantification, and timing, of manufacturing and associated operations.

A precise definition of a general 'staff-officer' role which included each of these three categories was evolved, and distinguished from operational roles. It was suggested, moreover, that the division of the planning and control of manufacturing activities into these three dimensions was a specific example of a more general proposition: that all work has three dimensions – the *personnel*, the *technical* and the *programming*. Further it was suggested, inherent in the organization of any large or complex operational process is the possibility of establishing three staff-officer roles each concerned with one of these three dimensions of work to help the manager ultimately accountable for the totality of operations.

Returning to hospitals, it has been possible to identify certain existing roles which conform closely to the general Glacier-definition of staff officer, though whether or not they fit into one of the

[12] Sometimes referred to in nursing spheres as 'acting-up'.

[13] See Brown (1960, Part IV). The general notion of staff-officer is of course much older than the Glacier Project, and emanates from military usage. (See Dale & Urwick (1960) for a general discussion.)

three categories of 'personnel', 'programming' and 'technical' is not so clear.

One clear example of staff-officer roles in hospitals arises in nursing, where senior nurses are regularly established in large hospitals with the main job of allocation of learner nurses to service departments, together with various subsidiary jobs in the recruitment, welfare, and in-service training field. The nurses in such roles are not the superiors (as here defined) of heads of service nursing areas, but they certainly do have some degree of authority to make their plans and programmes 'stick'. A generalized definition of the staff-officer role involved here may read as follows:

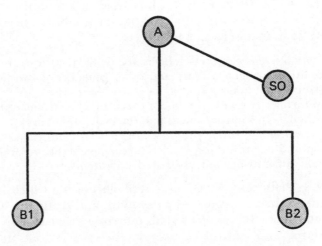

A superior (A) may need assistance in planning and co-ordinating the activities of his subordinates (B1, B2). Such assistance may be needed on personnel and organizational matters, on the programming of activities and services, on the techniques to be employed and perhaps financial matters. The superior may establish in any of these dimensions a subordinate role whose occupant has authority to interpret the superior's policy to his other subordinates and to give instructions within that policy. Such a role is called a *staff officer*. The relationship between the staff officer (SO) and other subordinates (B1, B2) is called a *staff relationship*.

If B1 does not agree with the staff officer's interpretation he cannot disregard it, but must take the matter up with A. A remains accountable for the work of B1 and B2 and the staff officer.

Returning now to the content of 'deputy' and 'assistant' roles, one evident possibility is that the titles might conceal in certain cases regular and straightforward staff-officer work in some special field as illustrated above. Or again, deputies and assistants might act as 'general staff officers' to the superior concerned, helping to form, and then to implement, policy in any field of the operational work to be managed. Or again, deputies and assistants act as high-level supervisors of those carrying out the operational work – a role which can scarcely be distinguished perhaps, from the 'general staff officer'. Or still again, deputies and assistants might in certain cases be found to be carrying full managerial accountability for certain operational areas.[14]

The main finding here then, is that whilst precise and usable definitions can be found for roles such as 'staff officer' and 'supervisor' and for the function of deputizing, no one general definition of the full-time role of deputy or assistant has yet been evolved.

Roles in Dual-Influence Situations

Another common feature of hospital organization, no doubt deriving from the peculiar mixture of many levels (hospital, group, region) with many disciplines (nursing, engineering, administration, etc.) is the frequent occurrence of roles in what may be described as 'dual-influence' situations.

Thus, H.M.C. officers are employees of the H.M.C., but they are also to some extent subject to the influence of their counterpart officer at regional level. Departmental heads at hospital level are subject to the influence of group heads in their particular occupation (where they exist) as well as to the influence of local administration. The work of ward housekeepers is controlled in part by officers of the domestic service, and in part by the nurses in charge of the wards concerned, and so on.

It rapidly became evident in the research that no one division of functions, no one set of characteristic role relationships, would adequately describe or adequately suit every hospital situation of this kind. In the attempt to distinguish the varieties of possibility

[14] Packwood (1971) provides a fuller, article-length, examination of these possibilities from the viewpoint of the Brunel Health Service Organization Research Unit.

here, we have evolved what may be called a 'profile-analysis' approach.

Such an analysis starts from the list of extended managerial functions described above. Discussions can be held with the person in the dual-influence situation, with his 'functional head' and with his 'local head' to establish common agreement as to how, requisitely, each of these managerial functions should be allocated – whether it should be allocated to the functional head or the local head, or shared between the two. Noting the answer against each item of the list provides in total a requisite 'profile' for that particular situation.

Statistically speaking, an astronomical number of alternative profiles is possible. In reality only a very limited number of combinations appear to make good sense as possible alternatives. Four[15] such possibilities are shown in Table 4.1. They may be described as:

(a) outposting (or local monitoring and co-ordinating);
(b) attachment (or co-management);
(c) functional monitoring and co-ordinating; and
(d) secondment.

A broad progression is discernible in this list from the one extreme (outposting) where the maximum influence or control rests with the functional head, to the other (secondment), where the maximum influence rests with the local head.

Outposting arises where some department is responsible for providing a service on a physically remote site. The staff of the department may be literally 'service-giving' as defined above, to the local site head, or they may be working collaterally with him. In either case, the local site-head carries in fact both a monitoring and co-ordinating role. He co-ordinates the work of the department to the extent that co-ordination is needed with other local departments, and he monitors the adherence of the staff of the department to any local policies and practices. In this situation, however, the outposted staff are definitely accountable only to

---

[15] Even these four may be too may. Outposting and secondment are clearly distinct. Functional monitoring and co-ordinating may possibly be an inappropriate (though extant) variant of attachment.

Table 4.1 Division of Managerial Functions in Dual-Influence Situations

Managerial Functions	Outposting (Local monitoring and co-ordinating).		Attachment (Co-management)		Functional Monitoring and Co-ordinating		Secondment	
	Function Head	Local Head	Function Head	Local Head	Function Head	Local Head	Function Head	Local Head
1. Participation in selection for role	o		o		?	o	o	o
2. Provision of induction, exposition of duties/policies	o	o	o	o	o	o	o	o
3. Exposition of techniques	o		o		o			o
4. Exposition of tasks and programmes, assignment of resources	o		o		o			
5. Help with work problems	o	o	o	o	o o	o o		o o
6. Reviewing performance	o	o	o	o	o o	o o		o o
7. Formal personal assessment	o		o		o	o	o	o
8. Providing or arranging training	o		o				o	o
9. Initiating transfer or dismissal	o		o		o	o	o	o

o – function carried out by one head only
o o – function shared between both heads

their functional head. He selects them, assesses them, and applies sanctions if needs be.

Attachment arises where the local head needs and is given a stronger controlling role. The member of staff concerned is not just 'outposted' by his functional head, the latter 'attaches' him to the local head. Both now share in selection, in assessment and in sanctioning – there is a joint-management situation. The local head will normally allocate tasks in keeping with local operational needs, and the functional head will normally be concerned with technical, training and organizational matters. If however the functional head does need to allocate tasks directly to the attached subordinate, he may do so provided it is understood that the latter will refer conflicting task-priorities for resolution to his operational chief.

Functional monitoring and co-ordinating marks a movement to a still weaker role for the functional head. Here, the local head alone selects, assesses, sanctions. Inevitably, accountability for the work of the subordinate now rests more firmly with the local head, and him alone, than it does in the case of attachment. However, it is still the job of the functional head to make sure that the work of the subordinate conforms to general policies established in the functional field concerned, and to co-ordinate developments specifically in this field.

In *secondment*, which implies a limited period of operation, with some definite point of termination, the functional head (the term 'functional' here is hardly in fact appropriate) loans his subordinate to the full managerial control of another (local) head for a certain period of time. What the first head retains is the right to join in the selection of the person to be transferred, in the first place, and a right to initiate his re-transfer, if necessary, at a later point. He retains also a continuing duty to consider the training and career needs of the seconded individual and therefore a need to carry out long-term assessment of him, to which the assessment of the local head is adduced in evidence. (Formal definitions of *outposting*, *attachment* and *secondment* are reproduced in Appendix A. A tested and agreed definition of *functional monitor-*

ing and co-ordinating, over and above what is described here, does not as yet exist.)

Representative Roles

All the kinds of roles considered so far have one thing in common. It may be assumed that all are part of a network established to put into practice the objects and policies established by some governing body. Each role is *executive* in character, and all together form an *executive role-system*, the prime 'work-doing' part of hospital organization.

However, certain other roles and role-systems may be discerned in hospitals which are not executive in nature, although they may on occasion become quite explicit and well-institutionalized. These are *representative roles* and *representative role-systems*.[16]

In general terms, the job of the representative is to voice the opinions and interests of the group or body who appoint him, in any communication or discussion with other groups or representatives. The mechanism of his appointment may be that of election by some group, or of appointment by some existing organized body. In carrying out his job, he will need freedom to interpret the views and interests of his constituents, or parent body, but how much freedom he is allowed and what limits he is set will vary from situation to situation. Lastly and most importantly, whatever other executive role he may also carry, as a representative he will be accountable only to those who appoint him and set his terms of reference.

Thus, elected chairmen of medical staff committees must be considered accountable in their dealings with hospital authorities to the consultants who elect them, and not to these authorities, even where they are, in another manifestation, in contract with these authorities. In the same way the elected spokesman of learner-nurse groups which exist in many hospitals are accountable in this role to the group, and not to the nursing administration. And where officers or members of local authorities conduct business as officers or members, they are accountable to their local authority committee, in contrast to the situation where they are

[16] For a further general discussion of representative systems in organization, see Newman & Rowbottom (1968, Chapter 7). See also end of chapter – Note 3.

carrying a second role, as members of health authorities appointed by a higher health authority, or by the Secretary of State – see later discussion.

Where a complex of representative roles emerges – as in hospital Joint Consultative Councils,[17] or in the interaction of various elected chairmen of separate medical committees – then a new kind of role-structure emerges with properties which can be sharply distinguished from the executive role-system alongside which it operates.

Types of Role-Structure in Hospitals

As far as internal organization is concerned, then, the *institutionalized* role-structures of hospitals are of three kinds – governing bodies, their executive systems, and (in varying degrees) representative systems which give vent to the reactions of particular groups within the executive systems (Figure 4.2).

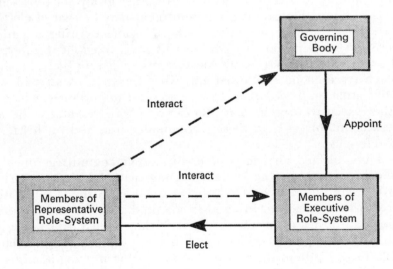

Figure 4.2

In exploring the detailed role-structure within each of these three, we have found certain common types of sub-system.

[17] See Miles and Smith (1969).

(1) *The Executive Hierarchy (Managerial Hierarchy).* This is the role-structure that arises from a succession of straightforward superior-subordinate (or managerial) relationships. Since it arises only within executive systems, it may without restricting its definition be called the executive hierarchy – though executive hierarchies are not the only component of executive systems. Final authority rests with the heads of the hierarchy. (See end of chapter – Note 3.)

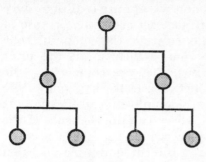

(2) *The Coalition or Collegiate.* This is a role-structure in which a number of people attempt to co-operate freely, without any of them having authority over the others, and without any authoritative external role to act as arbiter in cases of dispute. Action on significant issues can only proceed with the agreement of all, where the interests of all are involved. Meetings of members of the coalition thus have inevitably, a certain underlying element of negotiation.

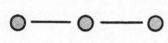

(3) *The (True) Committee.* This is a particular form of coalition, where it is agreed that action on disputed cases can be taken by *majority* decision, if unanimity cannot be reached. This presupposes some strong basic consensus of interest of members, and usually means that they have been elected or appointed by the same group or body in the first place.

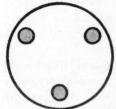

Executive hierarchies are found in hospital organization, for example, in nursing and in most departments below (and including) the level of departmental head – catering, domestic, engineering, etc. Pure coalitions arise in the interactions with hospital doctors and general practitioners, and between hospital authorities as a whole and local authorities. Something close to pure coalitions is found in the interactions of consultant medical staff, although employing authorities may in fact arbitrate on allocation of resources. The situation of chief officers of governing bodies at various levels is not quite intra-hierarchical – since there is often no one clear-cut managerial role – nor one of pure coalition, since the relevant governing body can in fact act as arbiter in case of disputes. Further clarification of the nature of the composite role-structures in these last two cases must clearly await the prior clarification of the elements of which they are composed – the relationships of consultants and chief officers to their employing authorities. The governing bodies of employing authorities are usually 'pure' committees, though where certain elements of the membership are appointed by other groups, as in the case of Executive Councils (see Chapter 2) a mixed committee/coalition constitution is implied (see later discussion).

Conclusion

To recapitulate, the aim of this chapter has been to summarize the main types of institutionalized roles and role-structures in hospitals which have so far been discerned as a result of discussion within the project. The definition of each which has evolved from these discussions, is not purely in terms of what 'exists' in some or other real-life position in the hospital world, but in terms of parti-cular 'packages' of characteristics of functions, authority and accountability, which are seen as serviceable and consistent by those with whom we have worked. Each definition refers to one unique set of characteristics. Where a range of significant options becomes discernible, the principle has been to attempt to dis-tinguish and separately identify the variants concerned.

Together, these definitions constitute a set of building-blocks in terms of which various alternative models of hospital organiza-tion (and indeed, as will be seen later, health service organization) may be constructed, considered and tested. Part II explores various major existing components of hospital organization in these terms.

There is no one magic answer to the right structures of inter-relationships for those working in hospitals. More than a dozen different kinds of basic relationships have been explored and defined here, each appropriate in its own situation. Without doubt, others will need to be added as the exploration proceeds. Nor is there any one kind of appropriate macro-structure – hierarchy, coalition, committee, or whatever – which is right for the whole organization. It might be agreed that the real task is to find the combination of those organizational elements in each health service situation which gives the optimum chance of efficient management, sensitivity to the needs and opinions of particular communities, and sensitivity to the needs and opinions of the various occupational groups employed within the service. (See Note 4 to this chapter.)

Notes to Chapter 4

Note 1. The Determinants of Requisite Organization (page 42)

The view of requisite organization as depending on the tasks to be carried out, the technologies and programmes employed, the environment to be worked in, and the characteristics of the people and other resources available, has obvious parallels with Lawrence and Lorsch's 'contingency theory' (Lawrence and Lorsch, 1967). However we must agree with Silverman (1970) that first and foremost it will depend on these things as they are perceived and interpreted by the *actors* in the situation (as long as we take care to include central government and local governing bodies as actors, and important actors at that). 'Organizations do not react to their environment, their members do. People act in terms of their own and not the observer's definition of the situation' (page 37).

Note 2. Style and Structure (page 45)

A large section of management and organization theory has in fact concentrated on appropriate managerial style – a social-psychological approach in contrast to the analysis of basic role-structure being undertaken here. Likert's 'overlapping work groups' (1961), McGregor's 'Theory X and Theory Y' approaches (1960), Blake and Mouton's 'grid' of production-oriented or people-oriented managerial styles (1964), all attend basically to the style of human relation preferred by supervisors and managers, and to the social atmosphere they attempt to create. On the whole, the earlier work was dedicated to the view that participative, democratic styles always scored over authoritarian or directive ones. Later writers (Fiedler 1966, Reddin 1970) suggest, more plausibly perhaps, that different styles are appropriate in different situations. For hospitals, it is interesting to note that Revans (1969) and his colleagues, investigating nurse-student wastage, found no evidence to suggest one way or the other that this was connected with how authoritarian an attitude was held by ward sisters with whom student nurses were in contact (page 73). Indeed, Revans correctly discerns just the distinction being made here between managerial functions and authority on the one hand, and managerial style on the other when he observes

'a system of authority seems to be as necessary for the student nurse to accept as it is for the matron and ward sister to exercise; the question for us is of the spirit with which the system of authority is informed'. (Page 68).

But the distinction is by no means universally recognized, Hunter (1967) in advocating the replacement of 'hierarchical' organization by 'arena' organization with such characteristics as 'control from within (the individual)' 'interlocking-roles' 'a philosophy of getting things done' and 'generation of an atmosphere of mutual trust' is surely bringing style and role structure into hopeless confusion.

Note 3. Executive and Representative Systems (page 63)

Consideration of 'executive' and 'representative' roles does not exhaust the variety of possible ways of interpreting the infinitely complex behaviour of individuals in organizations in terms of role-concepts. Any social-psychological approach might employ quite different terms for describing the roles played by particular individuals in particular group-encounters: to take one example more or less at random, Bales' 'task specialist', 'social specialist', 'overactive deviant', and 'underactive deviant', or 'scapegoat' roles (Bales 1966). Our study is concerned with roles that have been, or may readily be, institutionalized. So that their characteristics exist over periods of time, independently of the particular performers who fill them. So far all the institutionalized roles which we have identified have been describable in one or other of the executive categories listed above, or as representative, or as associated with some governing body.

Note 4. Hierarchy and Bureaucracy (page 65)

Note that 'hierarchy' is being used in a precise and restricted sense here, as a succession of superior-subordinate relationships, where again superior-subordinate is being used in a defined sense, excluding for example the relationships between a governing body and its officers and appointees, or between a governing body and a subordinate governing body. Nor should hierarchy as used here be equated with the more general notion of bureaucracy. Mouzelis (1967, page 53) has amply demonstrated the confusion and ambiguity about the way this later concept is used in modern social theory.

In particular 'hierarchy' as used here does not necessarily imply the proliferation of paper, rules or regulations, or the imposition of an authoritarian, hide-bound managerial style. There is certainly no assumption as to how much or little discretion subordinates are allowed in carrying-out their work (Mouzelis, page 41), although the myth of the totally-regulated work organization is not accepted.

Part II
Patterns of Existing Hospital Organization

5 Organization of Medical Staff

In Part II we shall be describing the results of studying and analysing organization and organizational problems in collaboration with various groups of staff – medical, nursing, paramedical, and administrative – using the terms and elements of description described in Part I. Together these results combine to produce a tolerably broad picture of the patterns of existing hospital organization in all its parts. Let us start with work on medical organization.

Generally speaking, the position of doctors in hospitals presents a fascinating, and possibly unique, situation to any student of organization. Never have so many highly influential figures been found in such an equivocal position – neither wholly of, nor wholly divorced from, the organization which they effectively dominate.[1] Formally employees of the hospital authorities, many clearly do not primarily think of themselves this way, and conceive 'the hospital' as some separate entity to which they may or may not happily relate.[2] It is, perhaps, not so surprising that the expressed attitude to the hospital and its staff (and the hospital staff's attitude to them) so often reflects this ambivalence.[3]

[1] This comment refers, of course, to the British scene. Nevertheless, there is manifold evidence of its applicability too in the U.S.A. See Smith (1958), Perrow (1965), Freidson (1970).

[2] In sociological language, their orientation is professional rather than bureaucratic – see end of chapter, Note 1.

[3] These comments would apply more to some doctors than others: for example, consultants in general rather than junior medical staff; and particularly part-time consultants rather than full-time ones, or those, in fact, running substantial hospital departments. Nevertheless, the common attitudes show themselves: 'you have to remember', said one consultant 'that the hospital is only there to help the doctor treat his patients'. Complaints of 'bureaucracy', 'red-tape', 'inefficiency' amongst 'them' (the adminis-

Looking back on discussions over the last three years[4] the issues that have arisen over the position of medical staff fall into three main groups:

(1) *The clinical autonomy of the hospital doctor.* Doctors by their powers of admission, prescription of treatment, and discharge, vitally affect all current expenditure in hospitals. Moreover, their actions and attitudes determine to a large degree the final quality of the service received by patients. How much freedom do they need to do their job properly? Can one discern the limits of this freedom? What control of their work is possible and desirable, and who should exercise it?

(2) *The authority of the hospital doctor in relation to his various hospital colleagues.* The questions here follow closely from those above. What is the authority of the hospital doctor in relation to other hospital doctors of various grades, in relation to nurses, physiotherapists, administrators, general practitioners, etc.?

(3) *The relationship of the hospital doctor to the management of the hospital.* Following on again: to what extent does or may the individual doctor play a managerial role? What mechanisms allow him and his medical colleagues to participate fully in the management of their own hospital, or of the service as a whole, and (turning the question around) to what extent is it possible for doctors as a group not only to manage, but be managed by, those who have responsibility for provision of the total service?

Each of these three groups of questions will be considered in

---

tration in general, but never in particular – see Anderson et al, 1971) are legion. Needless to say, this attitude is often reciprocated. 'The thing is to get control of the doctors,' says one administrator. 'The rest don't matter. You can't do it too openly, you've got to build up your position over time.' 'No use talking to us about good management,' say the nurses. 'Talk to the doctors – they are the ones that so often put a spoke in the wheel.'

[4] Up to the autumn of 1971 we have completed intensive field-discussions with sixty consultants (from five hospital groups), eleven junior hospital doctors of various grades (from three hospital groups) and seven general practitioners (from three hospital groups). In addition, project-formulations have received discussion and testing in four three-day research conferences, each involving about a dozen consultants from a number of different hospital groups in the N.W. Metropolitan Region, and from a wide range of specialisms. To these must be added, of course, innumerable discussions we have had with senior administrative and nursing staff about the position of doctors.

turn in this chapter. In relation to the first two groups, a substantial amount of well-tested field material has been assembled. Discussions about the third area – the place of doctors as a group in the hospital service as a whole[5] are at a much earlier stage, and the conclusions here are, therefore, more tentative.

The Clinical Autonomy of Consultant Staff

One interesting feature of many earlier discussions with consultants was the way that, as a researcher, one regularly felt oneself to be off the track, to have lost rapport, if questions were posed such as: 'to whom are you accountable in the service?' or 'who sets your duties and tasks?' Ambiguous answers to the first question would be received like: 'I am responsible in the end only to my patients, (or) my colleagues, (or) my profession, (or) myself.' Answers to the second were less ambiguous: 'Nobody!'

Subsequent project work in one area produced the following agreed statement of the basic duties of a consultant, ignoring for the moment any departmental or administrative responsibilities he might have.[6]

The Basic Duties of a Consultant

For a 'clinical' consultant, i.e. one who carries responsibility for the treatment of patients.
  (1) To examine patients and record information of their condition.
  (2) To treat or prescribe treatment for patients.
  (3) To give advice to colleagues on request on cases referred to them.
For an 'advisory' consultant i.e. one whose work is to provide advice on request to clinical consultants.
  (1) To give advice to colleagues on request, on cases referred to them, in the light of such investigations as may have been carried out.

[5] The meat, for example of 'Cogwheel' discussion ('Cogwheel' Report 1969).
[6] This particular project involved fourteen consultants from a wide range of specialties (including surgery, general medicine, radiology, pathology) who worked together in one large hospital. General statements of roles were produced in collaboration with each consultant. The results were summarized and compared, and a general statement was finally produced and agreed after a series of discussions with a special sub-committee of the medical staff committee of the Hospital formed for this purpose.

For all consultants.

(1) To comply with certain legal procedures (e.g. issuing death certificates and cremation certificates) on appropriate occasions.

(2) To provide the referring doctor with information about his patient.

(3) To give professional training to junior medical staff who work with him.

Now it may be observed that these duties have a particular character. They are not of the kind that are delegated to the consultant by some more senior officer of the service. Nor are they commonly specified in this detailed form in contracts of employment. In fact, contracts usually specify little more in this regard than the name of the specialty which the consultant is to pursue – 'general physician with a special interest in gastro-enterology' for example. These duties arise not by virtue of the consultant's membership of a particular hospital, but at a more basic level, by virtue of his membership of the profession or a particular branch of it. They are duties which come primarily from, and are defined primarily by, a professional role, rather than from a role in a particular executive system.

What degree of discretion accompanied these professional duties? In the same project the precise area of clinical or professional discretion of the individual consultant was agreed to be as follows:

(1) Deciding in all matters to do with the treatment of individual patients – priority of examination or treatment or advice, clinical investigations necessary, form of treatment, referral to other consultants, referral to medical social workers, admission to hospital, outpatient examination, discharge, optional post mortems; also, when to decline a request to see a patient because the disease is outside his area of competence or because he has insufficient time to make a true appraisal of it.

(2) Deciding what clinical information to record in patients' records, to communicate to the patient, to hospital staff or to the referring doctor;

(3) Deciding what training to give to junior medical staff.

(4) Deciding what clinical research or development work to undertake, and what time to devote to further personal professional development through reading, visits, attendances at conferences and lectures, etc.

(5) Deciding what work to carry out on hospital or professional working parties or committees (as invited).

(6) Deciding when to accept invitations to lecture to nurses (although specific contracts to do this sort of work are sometimes made).

Again, this discretion was not seen as *delegated* discretion, in the way, for example, that discretion is delegated by principal officers of the service to their assistants. Where discretion i.e. authority, is delegated by a superior, it may be retracted or modified by that superior at some later stage, if he wishes. But consultants did not see themselves as subject to any superior who could assign or retract authority in any way – they saw themselves as having definite and positive discretion in these matters – as having *autonomy*, in fact. Assuming that no freedom is limitless, what are the limits of this autonomy? The sum of these and many other project discussions to date suggests the following general answer. The freedom of the consultant is subject to three main groups of constraint:

(1) the norms of professional conduct;
(2) civil and criminal law;
(3) the conditions implicit in his contract –
    (a) implicit minima on the quantity and quality of work to be carried out (number of sessions attended, patients seen, etc.),
    (b) implicit minimum standards of general behaviour.[7]

Whether or not these are firm limits may be tested in each case by seeing the machinery that can call the consultant (or any other hospital doctor) to account and, if necessary, apply sanctions to him, should he overstep the limit. The machinery of law is obvious enough – hospital doctors, like all other citizens, may be charged with criminal offences or sued in civil actions for alleged negligence in carrying out their work. Final machinery in cases of professional misconduct is that of the Disciplinary Committee of the General Medical Council, where the ultimate sanction is that of removal from the Medical Register, with consequent termination of contract by the employing hospital authority. Procedures also exist whereby the employing hospital authority may (on medical

---

[7] Of course, too, the consultant is subject to the limits of the resources made available to him, but then this applies to everyone, in whatever work they do. This particular limit is perhaps best thought of as limit on existent *power*, rather than a limit on legitimate *authority*.

advice) act to prevent harm to patients resulting from the physical or mental disability of hospital doctors (defined in Ministry of Health Circular HM (60) 45), or act in cases involving personal misconduct, professional misconduct, or professional incompetence (defined in Ministry of Health Circular HM (61) 112). The employing authority, too, could clearly terminate a consultant's contract where he was in flagrant breach of it, for example, regularly failing to attend sessions without any good reason.

Provided, however, he stays within these various limits, as will normally be the case, the consultant is accountable to no one for the way he exercises his freedom – for the decisions he makes. Hence the characteristic answers to the questions described above. Under normal circumstances the situation of having somebody armed with sanctions making a critical review of his work is unknown to the hospital doctor once he achieves consultant status. This is not, though, to say that he no longer feels responsibility – to keep the distinction between accountability and sense of responsibility made in Chapter 3 – both to his patients and to his fellow professionals. One prominent characteristic of his professional training is the way it tends to strengthen this feeling of responsibility and 'inner-direction', to encourage him to 'internalize' professional and ethical standards.[8]

Why is the consultant in this enviable but demanding position? Two possible answers occur.[9]

[8] See for example the description of professional training from this point of view in Merton et al (1957) *The Student Physician*. However, Freidson (1970) argues strongly of doctors in general that it is not sufficient to rely merely on professional training and professional socialization to safeguard the quality of medical care to the community. He argues for the desirability of formal periodic reviews by doctors of the work of their fellows, fortified by sanctions, as well as for other mechanisms of external control.

[9] We have already received criticisms that our approach is too conservative, too concerned with the *status quo*, and never more so than our complete refusal to question the power and dominance of doctors within hospitals. Such criticisms miss the point. It is not part of our chosen role to take a stand as observers in criticizing the present or any other distribution of power in hospitals. Indeed we are not directly concerned with *power*, as such at all; we are concerned with *authority*, and with questioning (with our clients) what makes this or that degree of authority desirable or legitimate. In this case, the question is, what objective facts of the situation (social or technical) justify the apparent complete authority of consultants to determine treatment, within broad and fixed limits?

The first relies on the conventional analysis of profession. (See end of chapter – Note 2.) One of the central attributes of the developed profession is specialist knowledge – a knowledge that can be usefully applied only by the practitioner and which it is impossible even for the most intelligent layman to grasp and apply in full. (Hence also the necessity of leaving both research and training – the development and transmission of the special knowledge – to the profession itself.) Given this situation, the argument goes, only a professional can be in full managerial relationship to another professional, since the managerial relationship implies the ability to assess in total the work of the subordinate, and the ability to 'zoom-in' and guide that work when the subordinate runs into trouble.

There is little doubt that medicine, perhaps of all professions, has this body of esoteric knowledge at its core; but then this argument can be applied with varying strength to many other professions employed in the health service – physicists, engineers, architects, pharmacists and so on. A whole spectrum of 'professions' can be discerned, with varying degrees of density and difficulty of core-knowledge. Is there a dividing line between those which are susceptible to lay management, and those that are not; and if so, where does this line come?

An alternative explanation of the autonomy of the medical consultant turns, however, on another feature which does seem to differentiate medicine sharply from most, if not all, other hospital professions. This second explanation stresses the peculiar character of the personal bond between the doctor and 'his' patient, between the patient and 'his' doctor. As the practice of medicine has developed, at least in Britain, the patient entrusts himself, in all his vulnerability, to the care and direction of a personally-identified physician, and not to that of an impersonal agency.[10] The doctor may have assistants, but for the reassurance

[10] Two vivid accounts of the binding nature of the relationship between the doctor and his patient, quite different in kind but both outstanding in insight and sensitivity, are provided by Berger's half-biographical, half-impressionistic description of the life and work of a country doctor on the one hand, and Parsons' celebrated analysis of the professional role of the doctor and the 'sick-role' of the patient on the other. (Berger 1969, Parsons 1951, Chapter X.) Parsons emphasizes the functions of the various patterns of relationship between patient and doctor which have become institutionalized to cope with situations which are characterized:

of the patient he must be personally known to the patient, and visibly seen to be directing the course of treatment at his own discretion.[11] If the consultant were known to have a superior with full-managerial authority, he himself would no longer be seen as the directing physician. That role would pass to the new superior, and the consultant would now be merely an assistant to some 'super-consultant' (see end of chapter – Note 3). (This argument of course would apply more strongly, or at least more obviously, to the clinical consultant with his 'own' patient, than to the advisory consultant e.g. the pathologist, where personal link with the individual patient is less obvious).

Relationship of R.H.B. or Board of Governors to Consultants

Whatever the logic of either or both of these arguments, however, the fact of the matter is that the relationship of the R.H.B. (or Board of Governors) to the consultant whom it employs is at present far from a managerial one. The exact function of the R.H.B. appears to be as follows:

(1) appointing properly-qualified consultants, following professional advice;

(2) negotiating or re-negotiating specific contracts of employment with these consultants, to meet service needs as they change;

(3) providing (through the medium of the H.M.C. or directly) such resources of staff, equipment and facilities as they think fit, for the use of consultants;

(4) ensuring that consultants adhere to the conditions of their contracts.

(a) by the high anxiety of patients, and the real possibilities of permanent disability and death;

(b) by the peculiar inability of the patient to make objective appraisal of his own situation and needs;

(c) by the necessity for intrusion into the most private life, and even on occasions into the very person itself of the patient; and

(d) by the absence of complete predictability and control, even with the advance of medical science, coupled with the need to create and maintain an atmosphere of optimism and confidence.

See also the discussion of the doctor-patient relationship in Freidson (1970).

[11] Evans (1970) has pointed out that this argues for the possibility of a two-rank hierarchy in clinical medicine, but no more. This does in fact seem to be the case in practice – see later discussion in this chapter.

The R.H.B. has no authority to provide formal assessments of the ability of any clinical consultant, nor has it authority to award or withhold merit payments at discretion.[12] On the other hand, as mentioned above, the R.H.B. has the authority in the last resort to terminate contracts, having followed certain laid-down procedures, where consultants have seriously transgressed the boundaries of tolerable freedom.

In practice, much of the detailed execution of these functions is carried out in Regions by the Senior Administrative Medical Officer of the Region and his staff. Again, this officer is not the manager or superior of the individual consultant: his role might perhaps be described as a 'functional monitor and co-ordinator' in respect of hospital medical work throughout the Region.

The Relationship of the H.M.C. to Consultants

However, since it is within the hospital group that the consultant's work is actually carried out, it is at this level that the bulk of regular supportive and co-ordinating activity is required. The duties of the H.M.C. in relation to the consultant staff within its group were agreed by a number of consultants to be as follows: [13]

(1) participating in the appointment of individual consultants;
(2) providing certain facilities for consultants, e.g. premises, equipment, nursing, and other supporting services;
(3) ensuring that any complaints about medical staff made by patients or relatives are investigated;
(4) negotiating with consultants whatever changes they think necessary in the way in which, the place at which, or the time at which they (the consultants) make their services available;
(5) negotiating with consultants where they [i.e., the H.M.C.] consider that they may be making excessive demands on hospital services or incurring excessive expenditure on drugs and other medical materials;
(6) vetting proposals by consultants for increased medical establish-

---

[12] A system of merit-payments – which may add substantially to basic salary – does in fact apply to consultants. The arbiters are, significantly, fellow-professionals, members of a National Distinction Awards Committee appointed by the Secretary of State (see Ministry of Health Circulars HM 54 (109) and HM 55 (82) i.e. the judgement of *excellence* rather than *adequacy* of performance, is a professional matter, to be left to the peer-group.

[13] In the project with fourteen medical consultants, described above.

ment, for more beds, or for other new treatment facilities, before
passing them to the R.H.B. for approval (or approving the proposals themselves, where minor expenditure or new facilities can
be made out of H.M.C. funds);

(7) (in extreme situations) reporting to the R.H.B. any apparent
evidence of gross inadequacy or neglect on the part of any individual consultant.

Again, this is not a managerial relationship, but one which may
be described as both a monitoring and co-ordinating relationship,
and a sustaining relationship. Much of its detailed execution is
passed in practice to various senior H.M.C. officers – to the Group
Secretary, to the Treasurer (as regards monitoring of expenditure)
and to the (appointed) Medical Administrator, or (elected) Chairman of Medical Committee. The exact division of duties between
these various officers will no doubt vary from group to group.
In project-work with one appointed Medical Administrator[14, 15]
his administrative duties (as opposed to his representative duties
as Chairman of the Group Medical Advisory Committee, which he
was also) and the more significant authority available to him in
carrying them out, were analysed and agreed as follows:

(1) Ensuring on behalf of the H.M.C. that individual consultants or
'firms' of consultants have made all necessary arrangements to
provide a comprehensive provision of services in their various

[14] The particular Hospital Group concerned included only one large
hospital, the remainder being virtually 'cottage' hospitals, so that the fact
that this particular Medical Administrator carried a group role, rather than
a hospital role, was probably not of great significance.

[15] The general question whether there is a need for specifically 'medical'
administration, and if so, what is its exact content at various levels of the
Service, and who is to carry it out, is a large one. Various aspects of this
question are discussed in a number of places in the following pages. One
point about the use of the title 'Medical Superintendent' may however be
noted at this stage. This title was in common use in local authority hospitals
before nationalization, and still is in Scottish hospital groups, and in many
psychiatric groups in England and Wales. There is little doubt that in many
places at many times it has in fact implied a full-managerial role; not only
in relation to other medical staff in the hospital (who therefore might be
commonly thought of as assistant to the medical superintendent) but also
to nursing and administrative staff. With the growth and spread of the
individual specialist-consultant system, however, a managerial relationship
with medical staff becomes less and less possible (as argued above). The
title 'medical superintendent' may or may not remain, but the content
inevitably tends to change from managerial to monitoring and co-ordinating.

specialties, both for normal requirements and for round-the-clock emergency cover.

- He has discretion to decide how best to overcome evident deficiencies in medical services, by discussion and negotiation with medical staff.

(2) Ensuring that the best use is made of overall bed capacity in the face of fluctuating demands for various specialties.
- He has discretion to discuss and negotiate possible permanent changes in bed allocation with medical staff.
- He has discretion to authorize temporary transfer of beds from one specialty to another, in emergency situations.
- He has discretion to divert cases to other hospitals, in emergency situations.

(3) Providing answers to factual questions on medical matters posed by the H.M.C. or R.H.B. (for example, could the hospital take in cardiac patients with pace-makers).

(4) Participating as a full voting member in the appointment of all registrars and house officers, and advising on the appointment of other hospital staff, as required.

(5) Vetting and authorizing requests for 'contingency' items of medical equipment.

(6) Ensuring that good discipline is maintained in the Junior Medical Mess.

(7) Progressing, as requested, the provision of reports, or the payment of their fees where medical staff are making medical reports in legal proceedings.

(8) Investigating, and reporting on, all complaints concerning medical staff directed to him by the Group Secretary.
- He has discretion in deciding how best to explore the complaint with the medical staff concerned.
- He has discretion in deciding what personal view of the matter to express in his own final report.

(9) Attending H.M.C. Meetings to give information or advice on any of the above matters.

The main point to emphasize again, is that this is not the specification of a managerial role.

In field-work with the physician-superintendent of another group, somewhat the same kinds of functions emerged in a statement of role prepared with him. Again, he was clear, following analytical discussion, that his role was not that of an executive manager of his consultant-colleagues. Broadly his role was that of a co-ordinator, with authority to take decisions within policies agreed by his colleagues without constant reference back to them. He also saw himself as a 'spokesman' for his colleagues on some occasions, and on others as a communicator of messages to them from the hospital authorities.

Some Effects of the Lack of a Clear Concept of Autonomy, and its Limits

Given on the one hand general appreciation of the clinical autonomy of the individual consultant, but given also the common absence of any clarity on precisely what this autonomy includes, and where it ends, the situation described in the following extract from a project report[16] is perhaps not surprising.

> For administrative staff, difficulty lay in the fact that each consultant could independently approach whichever member of staff he thought most appropriate on any matter he wished to raise, there being no organization among medical staff to collate and select from their individual requests the most representative in any given sphere. Consultants therefore approached the House Governor, the Deputy House Governor, and Hospital Secretaries, as they thought best, a procedure that was time-consuming and made necessary much cross-informing to avoid confusion. Formulation of policy was made more difficult under these circumstances.
>
> Similar problems were found by senior nursing staff at CNO, PNO and SNO levels, who would be asked by consultants to provide services for which no policy existed, but initially on so small a scale that refusal would be unnecessary, although subsequently it might be found that demands were building up to quite considerable proportions, necessitating decisions on policy which might have been more useful if taken at an earlier stage.
>
> The problem of dealing with requests and suggestions from consultants and other medical staff was complicated by the feeling that such requests, sometimes, though not always, carried the force of instructions. Ward sisters felt that consultants had authority over them, for example. So also did paramedical staff, such as the dietitian. Administrative staff felt that requests from medical staff carried

---

[16] This particular report summarized discussion with a number of senior administrative and senior nursing staff in a teaching hospital group, and thus stresses their particular viewpoint. At that time, no work had been carried out with medical staff in the group to establish their view of the matter.

special weight. The relationship of the medical staff to the rest of the hospital was however not specified. Their authority over ward sisters was felt to differ from that of the PNO. Similarly, a consultant's request to a Hospital Secretary was felt to differ from the instructions he received from the House Governor. What these differences between medical authority and other authority were based on, and how they affected the relationships between medical and non-medical staff, was not known. The feeling that authority was one of the elements in the relationship added to the difficulty of keeping a clear view of the lines of executive authority.[17]

The problems of coping with the situation of 'creeping developments' diagnosed here has really two aspects:

(1) defining the exact authority of the consultant in his individual encounters, and
(2) evolving a better system for the integrated development and control of medical services as a whole, throughout the hospital.

Let us concentrate for the moment on the first, dealing with the relationship of the consultant to his fellows, to junior medical staff, to nurses, to administrative and paramedical staff, and to general practitioners.

Relationships of Consultants to Each Other and to Junior Medical Staff

In relation to each other, it will be obvious from what has been said above that consultants cannot carry managerial or supervisory authority. No consultant could give instructions on clinical matters to another without breaking the thread of the personal consultant-patient 'contract'. In an organizational sense, all consultants are basically equal, and form together what is essentially a large *collegiate-structure*, or *coalition* in any hospital in which they work.[18]

[17] H. L. Smith (1958) describes situations of the same kind frequently arising in American hospitals.

[18] Actually, the exact quality of interrelationships is not quite 'pure' colleague, i.e. without the possibility of any third-party arbitration; nor is it 'pure' collateral, i.e. subject to the general arbitration of a shared superior as described in Chapter 4. The exact relationship should perhaps be described as 'quasi-collateral'. There are many issues on which the 'cross-over point' – the employing authority – may not arbitrate, but there are

Having said that all consultants are organizational equals, one reservation must be made. It now begins to appear from project work that certain consultants are appointed or elected to carry some limited monitoring and co-ordinating role in relation to their fellows. This appears to be the case regularly in radiology and pathology. It may also cover the case of the 'senior consultant'; where two or more consultants of like specialty band themselves together into a 'firm'. It may possibly also fit, to some extent, the position of chairmen of various kinds of medical committees.

For example, in one project[19] a monitoring and co-ordinating role in the terms described below was seen for both:

(a) the 'head' radiologist in relation to the other two radiologists also employed in the hospital; and
(b) the 'chief' pathologist (a microbiologist) in relation to
 – the consultant in haemotology
 – the consultant in histology
 – the principal biochemist
 – the chief physicist

The agreed characteristics of this monitoring and co-ordinating role as stated in the final project-report were:

(1) The duty to ensure that agreed policies for change are put into effect, for example, for extension of services, or for new training arrangements for technical staff, or for introduction of new administrative procedures;
(2) the duty to monitor the adherence of fellow-consultants to agreed policies and procedures, and of drawing the attention of those concerned to areas where there is a danger of significant divergencies;
(3) the duty of collating all reports, proposals, and estimates, required for the department or group of departments, before onward transmission; subject to the right of other consultants

---

certain issues, for example any question of allocation of resources, and perhaps questions of trends of services to be provided, where they may. This is not to suggest that employing authorities do regularly decide, for example, how money for medical equipment is to be allocated between competing consultants, but it is to suggest that following independent medical advice they may always arbitrate on such issues in the last resort.

[19] The project was in fact concerned with the general position of doctors associated with paramedical departments and included in discussions a head radiologist, a chief pathologist, a histologist, and a director of physical medicine in one H.M.C. group.

to make independent submission where there are important differences of opinion on content or presentation which it has not been possible to resolve;

(4) the duty of helping to induct newly-appointed colleagues into their jobs and into the working situation.

The further statement was added:

This is clearly to be distinguished from a *superior-subordinate* relationship. The departmental head, or head of the departmental complex (e.g. pathology) is not accountable for the work of his fellow-consultants (or for the work of the Principal Biochemist in the case of pathology) and is not required to make a formal assessment of their ability. His authority to act in this monitoring and co-ordinating role will only be as strong as the consensus of agreement to the policies which he is trying to implement. In the ultimate, he has no right to deploy sanctions in relation to his colleagues, so that his work rests on persuasion rather than authority.

Turning to junior medical staff, the position is quite different. 'Junior medical staff' here includes senior and junior registrars, house officers, and medical and clinical assistants, the last category being general medical practitioners who work for specified sessions in hospitals, often in addition to their general practice. In spite of the fact that consultants in the Regions have contracts of employment with one authority (the R.H.B.) whilst many of their juniors have contracts with another (the H.M.C.), we have found solid confirmation both in Regions and in Teaching Hospitals that the relationships between the two are clear and straightforward superior-subordinate ones. The consultant is accountable for the work of his juniors in all its aspects, he may prescribe that work, and he provides formal assessments of the capability of the junior.[20]

---

[20] This finding is in direct conflict to the common hasty sociological assumption that the organization of all 'professionals', whoever they may be, tends to the *collegiate*. Students who have looked more closely, such as Goss (1963) have, of course, seen elements of bureaucratic, or more precisely, hierarchical structure in the working relationships of doctors in hospitals. Goss, in the American hospital-setting discerned what she described as an 'advisory bureaucracy' (with some similarity to Gouldner's 'representative bureaucracy' or Wilson's 'semi-bureaucracy'), with senior doctors having the right to direct in administrative matters and 'the right to give advice that subordinates (sic) are obliged to take under critical review' in professional matters. Our finding here is of course stronger; but then the American setting does not include the rigid distinction between consultants and general

On the other hand, the same managerial relationship is not duplicated within the ranks of junior medical staff themselves. The relationship of the registrar to the house officer appears to be that of a *supervisor*, not a *superior* (see Chapter 4). Both the registrar and house officer regard the consultant as their immediate boss.[21]

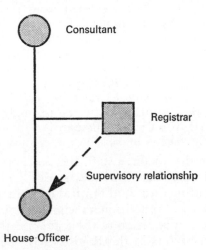

Figure 5.1

Relationship of Consultants and other Hospital Doctors to Nursing Staff

It is perhaps in the relationship of hospital doctors to nurses that the question where the authority of the doctors ends becomes most critical. By and large, in innumerable discussions of this issue with doctors, nurses and other hospital staff, this relationship has been recognized as a *treatment-prescribing* one, as defined in Chapter 4.[22]

This implies that *in regard to the treatment of the individual*

---

practitioners, and allows for the participation of medical practitioners of widely varying skill in the same hospital situation.

[21] This general conclusion was first suggested by a field-project involving all the members of a surgical team, including two consultants, a senior and junior registrar and two house surgeons. The general conclusion has since been tested and confirmed in many conference discussions.

[22] Certain possible exceptions to this general statement are discussed in Chapter 7 – The Organization of Nursing Staff.

patient the doctor may, in the end, prescribe what he likes in the way of treatments to be carried out, and services to be performed, in direct relation to that patient, given only that he keeps within the limits of what is lawful, ethical and professionally proper. (What can be *done* on the other hand, is subject, as in all things, to the iron law of availability of resources. Whether or not instructions, however legitimate, can be carried out in practice will always depend on the availability in the event of nurses, drugs, equipment, diagnostic facilities, etc. – but this is another matter.)

But where does this prescriptive right end? May the doctor also prescribe the way the ward or theatre or clinic is to be organized as a whole, and the services as a whole to be made available? The consensus of many discussions on these questions is that the doctor has not got prescriptive rights in these matters; that on these broader issues he ought to be regarded as in a negotiating, persuasive role, rather than an authoritative one.

If this is so then the doctor does not have the *right*, for example, to decide the layout or equipment of wards, to decide the general format of records to be kept, or the general pattern of nursing procedures to be adopted. He does have an obvious *interest* in these matters and may hope to persuade nursing staff to make the change he requires. On the other hand, he presumably does have, for example, the right to decide unilaterally if necessary the allowable visiting arrangements for one particular patient, the need of that patient for more or less privacy, the clinical data to be registered for that particular patient and the nursing procedures to be adopted for that patient – again noting the possible constraints on total resources available.

The general implication of this analysis is that whilst decisions on individual cases may be made unilaterally by the doctor, general policies on treatment and service provision should be a matter for bilateral agreement with nursing staff at ward or unit level, in the first instance. Again this leaves the question how, more generally, policies on medical services should requisitely be set and sanctioned within the hospital as a whole.

Relationship of Hospital Doctors to Administrative and Paramedical Staff

Similar issues obviously arise in the relationships of doctors to physiotherapists, occupational therapists, pharmacists, medical records officers, and other paramedical and administrative staff. In general, the same conclusion could be agreed; that where policy issues are concerned the discussion should be bilateral or multi-lateral, so that final decisions rest entirely on mutual agreement, apart from those questions on which the employing authority may act as 'cross-over point' arbiters. More detailed consideration of relationships with these groups of staff is given in the chapters that follow.

Relationship of Consultants to General Practitioners

The relationship between consultants and general practitioners who refer their patients to them is one in general unstructured by executive authority, and not (apparently) susceptible to the decisions of any governing body or council; but it is structured by certain expectations that have accrued in relation to professional behaviour. It is, for example expected that the consultant will keep the referring general practitioner properly informed of the progress of the case. It is expected that the consultant will not proceed to treat if the referring doctor specifically asks only for an opinion; but that the consultant may proceed to treat at his discretion as well as to diagnose, in many cases where the referring doctor may be assumed to be expecting this response. What seems certain is that the consultant has no authority, supported either by executive or professional sanctions, to prescribe the treatment to be carried out by the general practitioner. The relationship is one of referral and collaboration, not a treatment-prescribing one.

Where general practitioners have facilities to admit patients to hospital beds under their own medical supervision, in 'cottage' hospitals or in 'general practitioner' wards, special problems of relationship arise with consultants who may be invited to collabor-ate in the same cases. A project which considered the position of the general practitioner in this situation and his relationship to any associated consultants produced the following agreed formulation: [23]

[23] This particular project involved discussions with five general practi-tioners at two different cottage hospitals, and with five consultants who regularly worked also at these hospitals. There was general agreement on the statements quoted here, apart from the reservations of one consultant

The H.M.C. has no authority over general practitioners, individually or collectively. General practitioners admit, treat and discharge patients entirely at their own discretion.

Conversely, the H.M.C. has complete authority over resources to be placed at the disposal of general practitioners on the staff of its hospitals. These resources include staff, equipment, and number of beds to be made available. The hospital authorities can, if they wish, convert general practitioner beds to other uses or make policies about categories of patients to be treated in the hospitals. These decisions can be made without the consent of the general practitioners. The authority to decide bed use rests with the R.H.B.; decisions about categories of patients to be treated are made by the H.M.C. It was felt that it was necessary for the H.M.C. to have this authority since it accepts legal liability for patients treated in G.P. hospitals. (Consultant staff also affect through the Medical Advisory Committee the decision as to categories of patients to be treated.)

The general, though not unanimous, opinion is that only general practitioners have authority to admit to G.P. beds. Some cases may be admitted and consultants' advice sought subsequently (see below). Patients who have seen a consultant in outpatients may, ostensibly, be admitted by the consultant. In fact, they are admitted in the general practitioner's name, and his implicit agreement is presumed.

Surgical Inpatients. It is the responsibility of the general practitioner to ensure that the patient is fit for operation, although the anaesthetist or surgeon may also check the patient's condition. The general practitioner administers the pre-medication in accordance with the wishes of the anaesthetist and surgeon. The surgeon is accountable for the conduct of the operation. He is also accountable for post-operative treatment until such time as he (the surgeon) leaves the hospital. (One consultant says however – until such time as the patient is discharged.)

Medical Inpatients. Consultant physicians examine inpatients only on the specific request of a G.P. As in the case of post-operative surgical treatment outlined above, the consultant only advises about treatment. The general practitioner has full authority to decide this. As before, even if treatment is started immediately following the consultant's prescription, the implicit agreement of the G.P. is assumed and he may change the treatment if he deems it necessary.

Discharge. In all cases the final decision to discharge a patient

---

in those places specifically indicated. The nature of these reservations is such as to make one think again about the possibility of something above simple collaborative relationships, perhaps in line with Goss's concept of 'advisory authority' (Goss 1963).

rests with the general practitioner. Often, however, the practitioner would agree with the consultant who has been advising about the case a date when the patient would be fit for discharge. (Again, one consultant disagrees with this opinion, regarding the right of the G.P. to discharge as a delegated authority.)

Emergencies. Since the general practitioner alone is regarded by most medical staff as accountable for his patient in the cottage hospital he has to be contacted first in a case of emergency. At her discretion the nurse in charge may also contact the consultant, if the G.P. is unobtainable or if she considers the matter to be of so serious a nature that consultant attention will in any case be necessary. General practitioners have an emergency 'on call' system among the staff so that one of their number is always available. When on call they are mutually authorized to treat each other's patients.

The Place of Consultants in Hospital Management

We now return to the third topic identified at the start of the Chapter – the relationship of consultants to the management of the hospital as a whole, and to the general development of services within it.[24]

In one obvious sense, every consultant is involved in management to the extent that he has subordinate staff working for him. Most consultants do in fact have some junior medical staff subordinate to them, and some, in certain specialties (as will be suggested in the following chapter) may well be effectively in managerial relationships to very large groups of paramedical staff, running into many dozens in number. Here, the consultant is the managerial head of his own hierarchy.

The deeper issue, however, is by what means the individual consultant becomes related not only to the management of his own firm or department, but to the management of the hospital as a whole.

It would be fair to assert in general, that there are two main ways in which employees in organizations may participate in the

[24] The material of this concluding part of the chapter is not drawn so directly from field project-work as that discussed in earlier parts. Most of our field-work to date has been concerned with the role of the individual consultant in relation to the rest of the hospital. However, the analysis of some of the broader issues of medical organization discussed here has been tested to some degree in conference discussion – for example, within four three-day conferences involving some three dozen consultants from various specialties.

management of the organization as a whole. One is as individuals, interacting directly with their superiors, or with other senior officers of the organization, or even directly with the governing body of the organization, so as to affect policy-formation by individual advice, persuasion, and pressure. The other is through banding as a group, attempting to agree common views and policies and then attempting, again by advice, persuasion, and pressure, to influence policy formation, by means of elected representatives.

One characteristic of a managerial hierarchy, is that any subordinate has a clear opportunity to affect policy-formation through interaction with his superior. However, consultants are not part of a larger managerial hierarchy; true, they may interact individually with senior officers (Group Secretaries, medical administrative officers etc.) or even, clumsily, with employing authorities themselves (R.H.B., Board of Governors), but this may not be such a potent means of influence. At any rate, the second channel, interaction through groups and representatives, is of prime importance in medical organization, as is evidenced by the wealth of existent (and vigorous) medical staff and advisory committees.

Any gathering of consultants allows the performance of two functions. Firstly, through their own interaction and mutual agreement they may be able to co-ordinate their activities, exercise mutual constraint, and resolve how they are to share out what are inevitably limited resources. This is a self-governing activity. Secondly, they may be able to form and express a strong and coherent view on any matters of concern so as to influence the decisions of the R.H.B., Board of Governors or H.M.C. This is both an advisory and a polemical activity.

In neither case is any question of managerial authority involved. For the first function an elected chairman is needed to steer collective discussion, and for the second, an elected spokesman to interpret and convey collective opinion. The two will usually be the same person. If a particular consultant is felt to be stepping out of line with regard to say, expenditure on drugs, or demands for equipment, or use of unduly unorthodox clinical methods, he may be subjected to the collective pressure of adverse opinion of his colleagues, but he cannot be given an instruction backed by managerial sanction. If consensus on a certain issue is reached in such a meeting, then it may well be that the chairman thereafter carries a monitoring and co-ordinating role in relation to that policy, in the same way as that described above for medical 'heads' of services. He may see that practical steps are taken to introduce some agreed policy, and he may draw the attention of any colleague to his deviation from that policy – but all in the end depends on pressure of group opinion, and not on clear-cut managerial sanctions of recorded reproof or dismissal from post.

What is obvious, however, is that such an elected chairman cannot be accountable to the hospital authority for carrying out such monitoring and co-ordinating work, or indeed, for the general way in which he carries out his representative role in helping to shape policy by communicating opinion. Since the consultant group elect him, it is this group, if anybody, to whom he is accountable, and it is this group who will assess the adequacy with which he carries out his chairman's role. They will decide whether or not he warrants re-election.

The Overall Control and Co-ordination of Medical Work by the Employing Authority

However, the hospital authorities – the R.H.B. or the Board of Governors – do themselves have a duty to ensure that the activities of consultants are co-ordinated with one another as well as may be, and that they are all carried out within certain overriding limits. They must watch for any 'out-of-bounds' activity by consultants, of the kind discussed earlier in this chapter (personal or professional misconduct, gross neglect of duty etc.). More than this (and what is more important in practice), they must also watch for adverse trends indicated by such matters as lower bed-utilization, unusually high mortality rates, and higher drug bills.

Having established that the hospital authorities have no right to *direct* in this latter area – in the area of 'within-bounds' clinical autonomy – one is inevitably talking of a situation of pure discussion and persuasion. This is essentially then a *power* situation, where if there is disagreement the outcome is influenced on the one hand by the need of the hospital to keep consultants in a position in which they will happily give their best work, and on the other hand, by the need of the consultants to make sure that the hospital authorities are in the frame of mind to provide them readily with the resources and facilities which they need. Here the immovable object of clinical autonomy, meets as it were, the irresistible force of control of resources.

Given this duty, the main organizational question is, how is the governing body of the particular authority going to ensure that it is carried out? It cannot do all the necessary work itself, and if it relies on a medical co-ordinator who is elected by his fellow consultants, it cannot be sure that the individual so elected is suitable for this work by the standards of the governing body, nor can it hold such a person accountable to it for the work he does as a co-ordinator. The inevitable conclusion appears to be that if the governing body wishes to ensure that such work is adequately carried out, it must perforce appoint its own officers to do so.

Conclusion

It appears, then, that there is a need to distinguish three separate activities, all generally 'managerial' in character:

(1) the management in the strongest sense of medical work through superior-subordinate mechanisms;
(2) the mutual co-ordination and internal self-regulation of medical work through group-activity, and the accompanying expression of group-consensus through elected representatives; and
(3) the monitoring and co-ordination of medical work by appointed officers of the employing authority. (See end of chapter – Note 4.)

Generally, the main project-finding as regards organization of medical staff does confirm a common impression that the role of doctors in hospital organization is special. The autonomy of the clinician seems to be both factual and also requisite – given, that is, the common desire for personalized treatment within an independent professional relationship rather than within the impersonally-defined service of a treatment-giving agency. Linked directly with the notion of genuine clinical autonomy is, then, the impossibility of hierarchical organization, i.e. full management of medical work as described at (1) above, above the level (consultant or general practitioner) where full clinical responsibility rests.[25]

[25] Although in many hospitals the medical superintendent did in the past, and may still in some places, play such a full-managerial role in relation to his medical assistants.

However, what has been possible within the project is to begin at any rate to move towards a closer definition of this area of autonomy, and the desirable relationships and counter-balances, as it were, which it brings into play. In collaborating with those in the field, we have started as described above, to identify:

(1) the place where the unilateral authority of the doctor based on his clinical autonomy prevails, and the place where his relationship with other officers becomes properly one of free negotiation;
(2) the typical means by which he interacts with his peers in order to reach mutual adjustments and a shared consensus on collective action required;
(3) the typical means (i.e. by elected representative) by which shared needs and opinions are communicated to the managing organizations of the hospital; and
(4) the typical means (monitoring and co-ordinating roles) by which the employing authority regulates his work and endeavours to bring it into line with the work of others within the hospital, whether these roles be played by medical administrators, lay administrators or both.

Notes to Chapter 5

Note 1. Doctors and Hospitals – 'Professional' and 'Bureaucratic' Organization (page 73)

As Perrow (1965) points out, hospitals have been a constant source of interest to sociologists and organization theorists, because of their mixture of 'bureaucratic' and 'professional' elements. Are they to be thought of as a whole, as 'professional' organizations, as opposed to 'semi-professional' or 'non-professional' (Etzioni 1964, Chapter 8)? Are there two well-distinguishable kinds of authority at work in them, 'administrative' and 'professional' (Op. cit. Chapter 8)? Are they to be thought of as bureaucracies of a special kind, 'advisory bureaucracies' (Goss 1963)?

Here, we shall choose to emphasize the similarity of hospitals to other organizations. Like other organizations, hospitals have governing bodies with given objects set by some higher association, that establish executive systems and appoint staff – professional, semi-professional or other – to forward these objects. Again, we shall emphasize the organizational base of all authority exercised within hospitals. For example, doctors in hospitals do not carry authority simply because they are doctors, but because they are also accredited members of the service. (The question of the general authority of the doctors in society at large is another matter.) As Freidson (1970, page 131) points out, technical expertise does not in itself constitute authority, and institutional status is needed in addition.

What we shall be concerned with in this Chapter and elsewhere, is in discovering how 'profession' as a factor affects the requisite organization of various different occupational groups within what we have called the executive system.

Note 2. Profession and Professionalization (page 79)

The study of what constitutes a profession and of the process of the development of profession – 'professionalization' – is a major field in itself. Goode (1969) provides a central introduction. He comments that study of various statements of the characteristics attributed to various occupations in order to prove that they are professions shows considerable agreement, but abstracts two 'core or generating traits', a basic body of abstract knowledge and the ideal of service (page 277). He goes on to elaborate various dimensions. Jackson (1970) in another general introduction stresses too the common orientation of the professional to universal areas of deep personal concern – the health of the body and mind, spiritual welfare, personal liberty and so on; and the consequent generation of high mystique where practitioners move freely in areas normally taboo and private.

For the discussion in mind here we may draw attention to such commonly agreed characteristics of profession as:

(1) The existence of a body of knowledge at a scientific level.
(2) The knowledge is applicable – a *technology* exists.
(3) There is exclusive competence – the science and technology is accepted as beyond the 'lay' group (the esoteric element).
(4) Hence the profession itself must be responsible for the transmission and development of knowledge (training and research).
(5) Members subscribe to a prime ethic of service rather than self-interest, but at the same time, aim to remain independent of the value-systems of clientele (detached involvement).
(6) The profession controls entry and exit.

Many writers stress that no one general definition can be expected to exist of what distinguishes a profession from a non-profession, and that the reality in any general view is of a spectrum in which various occupational groups exhibit more or less conformity to characteristics like those listed above, and compete to establish greater professionalism with all its associated status. Nevertheless, whilst this view may be true in general the specific questions remain: at what points of the spectrum of emerging professionalism do important revisions of organizational structure become necessary? As we have seen above, medicine has certainly reached the point where hierarchical organization *outside* the profession is inappropriate. Have other health professions reached this point, or will they?

Note 3. Official Definitions of 'Consultant' (page 80)

Two published definitions of 'consultant' support the argument quoted above for the special organizational position of the consultant. The Platt Report (1963) says: 'A consultant is a doctor chosen by reason of his ability, qualifications, training and experience, to take full personal responsibility for the investigation and/or treatment of patients without supervision in professional matters' (para. 40).

The Godber Report (1969) offers:

'A consultant is a doctor appointed in open competition by a statutory hospital authority to permanent staff status in the hospital service after completing training in a specialty and, in future, being included in the appropriate vocational register; by reason of his training and qualifications he undertakes full responsibility for the clinical care of his patients without supervision in professional matters by any other person; and his personal qualities and other abilities are pertinent to the particular post'.

Elsewhere in the same report, the length and difficulty of the progression to this position of licensed autonomy is stressed. For instance, the mean average age of first appointment to paid consultant posts in England and Wales between 1963 and 1967 stayed rigorously in the band 38-39 years (Para. 17). That is, it is usually ten years or more after graduation, with further rigorous training and examination, before the aspirant consultant 'arrives'.

Note 4. Medical Administration and Medical Representation (page 95)

Given the distinction between medical representation and medical monitoring and co-ordination described above it is possible to see an important difference between the recommendations of the so-called 'Cogwheel' Report (Ministry of Health 1967) and the Brotherston Report (1967) on medical organization in England and Wales, and in Scotland, respectively.

The Cogwheel Report recommended the establishment of various medical 'divisions' including all consultants of like or related specialty and their juniors, who work together in a particular group of hospitals. The chairman of each of these various divisions, and a chairman of an executive committee composed of these various divisional chairmen, were in all cases to be *appointed* by the hospital authorities concerned. (This mechanism of appointment would of course be inconsistent with true representative roles.) Brotherston recommended the formation of similar divisions but with an *elected* chairman. 'If we regard the formation of divisions in the clinical specialties as a voluntary act undertaken by the staff of those divisions in order to further certain of their responsibilities and duties on a group basis, then it seems clear that they, and they alone, should determine who their spokesman should be' (Para. 50). On the other hand they doubted whether election might be appropriate in cases like laboratory medicine, radiology, or radiotherapy, or in certain other cases (Para. 51).

One general point to be made here is that if such divisional bodies are not seen by their members as a voluntary coming-together with an elected chairman to act as mouthpiece, then it seems very likely that the same members may want to engineer or retain a separate group activity which is of this kind. If for example, divisions were to be established with appointed chairmen, then the consultants concerned would be likely to want to meet separately, perhaps in a larger group with their fellows from other divisions, under the leadership of their own elected chairman.

Generally as regards the administration of medical work, the arguments have long raged about the need for administrators with medical qualifications at various levels of the service. Boards of Governors have tended not to employ full-time medical administrators as such at Board level. On the other hand, R.H.B.s have had well-established systems of medical administrators under a Senior Administrative Medical Officer. Scottish practice, as we have noted, has been to have a Medical Superintendent at large hospitals. English and Welsh practice has varied; Bradbeer (1954) examined the matter closely and recommended the appointment of medical administrators at hospital level (Para. 71) but not at Group level, where reliance was to be placed on medical advisory committees with their own elected chairmen (Para. 88). For sanatoria and mental hospitals they recommended the appointment of medical superintendents (Paras. 110-143) apparently with a managerial relationship to other residential medical staff.

6 Organization of Paramedical Staff

Definition of Paramedical Staff

One of the striking features of the hospital service is the extraordinary proliferation of occupations and professions to be found in it. The presence of doctors and nurses is obvious and expected. Administrators too, are well visible to the public eye, at least in the higher reaches of their profession, by virtue of their public relations role. But beyond doctors, nurses and administrators – the often-depicted partners in a system of so-called tripartite management[1] – stands a large band of further occupations – supplies specialists, architects, engineers, builders, domestics, caterers, dietitians, laboratory technicians, physiotherapists and many others.

For convenience, these members of the service may be thought of as falling into two categories:

(a) those (other than doctors and nurses) who are directly concerned in the diagnosis or treatment of individual patients;
(b) the remainder, who supply services of a more general nature to patients or to staff.

The organization of the second group – the engineers, builders, caterers, domestics, etc. – will be considered in a later chapter. In this chapter the organization of the first group, the *paramedical staff*[2] will be considered. This group includes:

[1] See Chapter 10 for doubts on the reality of tripartite management in practice.
[2] Note the difference between *paramedical staff* as defined here, and *hospital scientific and technical staff* as defined in the Zuckerman Report (1968). For a start, Zuckerman specifically excludes what he calls the remedial professions, e.g. physiotherapists, occupational therapists, remedial gymnasts

art therapists
audiology technicians
biochemists
cardiological technicians
chiropodists
clinical psychologists
dietitians
laboratory technicians
medical artists
medical photographers
medical social workers
occupational therapists
opticians
orthoptists
pharmacists
physicists
physiotherapists
radiographers
remedial gymnasts
speech therapists.

The Main Problem of Paramedical Organization

In both project-work in the field and in conference discussion about the role of paramedical staff,[3] two issues have come time and

and speech therapists. He also excludes 'clinicians'. Radiologists are classed as clinicians but pathologists are not. Radiographers are classed as scientific and technical. The Report admits the difficulty of finding a satisfactory criterion to distinguish 'scientific and technical' staff from others. (Paras. 1.4-1.6.) Some staff with medical qualifications are included in the scientific and technical category.

In fact, although the Report is ostensibly about organization, like so many other hospital reports, little is said of executive or managerial structure, the main emphasis being on improved career planning and improved career structure. This being so, a categorization strictly according to groups with a common training and career structure might perhaps have been more appropriate.

[3] The material in this chapter is based on intensive discussion in field-projects with the following categories of paramedical staff: one audiology technician, one art therapist, one biochemist, one chiropodist, three dietitians, three chief laboratory technicians, one medical artist, one medical photographer, two head medical social workers, one psychiatric social worker, five head occupational therapists, one ophthalmic optician, one orthoptist, three Chief Pharmacists, three physicists, three Superintendent Physiotherapists,

again to the fore:

(a) lack of clarity about who, if anyone, is accountable for the work of paramedical staff; and

(b) lack of clarity in many cases about the authority, if any, of doctors in relation to the work of paramedical staff.

Both issues are illustrated by the following extract from a project-report based on discussion with five heads of paramedical departments in a teaching hospital group:

> In the case of paramedical staff a further problem was experienced. ... This concerned the nature of the relationships between paramedical and medical staff and between the medical and administrative staff. Paramedical staff felt themselves accountable at the same time to medical staff, to the House Governor, and to the Hospital Secretary in whose hospital they occupied the role of head of department. It was difficult to sort out how these accountabilities were related and who their superior was. While it was apparent that consultants approaching the House Governor over matters of budget allocation, for example, could directly affect the running of paramedical departments in terms of staffing, extent and nature of services provided, techniques and development, paramedical Group Heads did not feel medical staff to be their executive superiors. At the same time they received few if any instructions from administrative staff. In this situation the absence of explicit statements of their accountability led to a feeling among Group Heads of not being clearly located in the organization.

Paramedical staff, perhaps more than any other hospital staff, tend to 'float' organizationally, as indicated in this illustration. This is particularly true of the many who work alone or in very small groups in hospitals – dietitians, chiropodists, medical artists, and so on. It is commonly believed that their work is controlled in some respects by doctors, and in others by administrators. When the issue is pressed, the statement is often produced that they are 'clinically accountable to doctors, and administratively to administrators'. In fact it is highly doubtful whether 'accountable to' here could be taken as meaning (as we have defined it here – Chapter 3)

---

two physiotherapists, three Superintendent Radiographers, one speech therapist. In addition, some dozens of paramedical staff have discussed their organizational situation in research conferences. Field-project discussions have also included associated consultants and administrators in many cases, as indicated below.

'assessed by, and likely to be sanctioned by'; or turning the proposition round, it is highly doubtful whether either doctors or administrators regard themselves as clearly accountable for the work of paramedical staff in many cases.

As in many areas of hospital work, there is a general feeling that if the quality of particular paramedical services becomes too bad a growing pressure of hospital opinion will somehow force eventual action – probably action by the administrators on the advice of the doctors. Until this point is reached, however, many paramedical staff are likely to be left much on their own.

Again, paramedical staff, finding themselves for the most part in small and relatively low-status groups (relative to doctors for example) tend to be left out of many important existing policy-forming bodies, and without policy-forming bodies of their own. In the absence of either a clear line of hierarchical authority, or the self-regulating bodies typical of medical organizations, opportunities for the systematic and positive development of paramedical services are therefore reduced. As one Chief Pharmacist indicated to us, his one chief and overriding organizational problem was to establish adequate links for ensuring that his department got its proper share of the annual budget.

Three Alternative Organizational Positionings for Paramedical Staff

As far as the accountability of paramedical staff is concerned, when one steps back to survey the possibilities broadly, three evident alternatives appear (discounting the reality, as discussed above, of 'clinical accountability' to a doctor, and 'administrative accountability' to an administrator as a fourth alternative):

(1) They may be situated hierarchically, under the management of a doctor.
(2) They may be situated hierarchically under the management of an administrator.
(3) They may be subordinate only to the governing body of the employing authority.

Furthermore, it might immediately be supposed, that were any member of paramedical staff in the position of an independent therapist, with his or her own personal patients or clients under treatment determined only by him, then the same arguments as applied to consultant staff would come into play. The therapist

concerned could not be part of any larger hierarchy, and would
have to be considered in direct contract with his employing authority, as in the third possibility above. He would be subject to
monitoring and co-ordinating activity, and no doubt some of this
activity would be delegated by the governing body to one of its
officers to carry out. In this particular case, we might immediately
say then, that the requisite position of the paramedical specialist
concerned would be as shown in Figure 6.1.

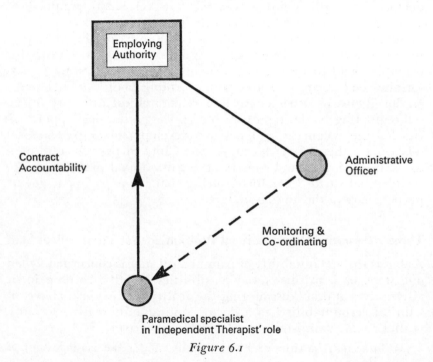

Figure 6.1

Further again, if the person concerned had colleagues in the same
specialty also acting as independent therapists, he would no doubt
group with them from time to time, in a meeting of equals to
discuss matters of mutual concern, much as consultants do.

Having sketched at least three major alternatives for the requisite positioning of paramedical staff in the organization, the
results of actual discussions as to which of the three possible answers
is requisite for various categories of paramedical staff will now be
described.

Paramedical Staff Hierarchically Organized under the Management of a Consultant

Work in a number of field-projects, confirmed in conference discussions, has suggested that the following large groups of paramedical staff are in most situations organized hierarchically under the management of medical consultants as illustrated below:

Consultant	Intermediate Management Level	Subordinates
Radiology	Superintendent Radiographer	Radiographers
Pathology (various branches)	Chief Laboratory Technician	Laboratory Technicians
Opthalmology	——	Opticians, Orthoptists
Otolaryngology	——	Audiology Technicians
Physical Medicine	Superintendent Physiotherapist	Physiotherapists
	Head Occupational Therapists	Occupational Therapists.

This organization is not only considered requisite by most people immediately concerned, but appears to be close to the extant situation in the places we have explored – though, as always, there is the difficulty of knowing what the 'extant' is until it is formulated, and once it is formulated and agreed as suitable by some criteria, the very statement of organization begins to affect behaviour and attitudes.

For example, in one field-project concerned with the organization of an X-ray department, the main outline of the structure was seen and agreed by all concerned[4] to be as shown in Figure 6.2.

The individual radiographers were seen in subordinate relationships to the superintendent radiographer, and the latter in turn subordinate to one radiologist, the one who had by custom (but not by specific arrangement) been regarded as 'chief' in the department. The other two radiologists were not in superior-subordinate

[4] Involved in the discussions, were three radiologists, the superintendent radiographer, and at a later point, the local Project Steering Committee of the Hospital Group concerned.

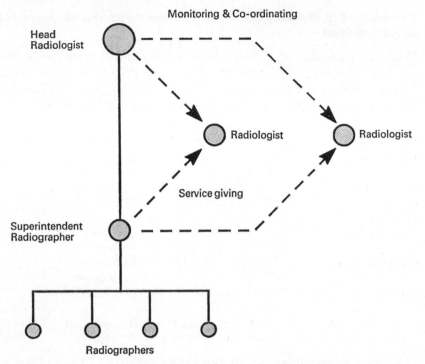

Figure 6.2   Organization of an X-ray Department

relationship to the superintendent radiographer, but could expect services from the radiographers on demand, in order to carry out their primary work which was to examine and report on films.

Although it was agreed that the chief radiologist was responsible for the general organization of the department, it was recognized that he was not the superior of the other two radiologists, and at the time of the initial project the relationship between all three was described as 'collateral'. In fact, in a later project (which involved of this group, only the head radiologist) the relationship was described as 'monitoring and co-ordinating' within the framework of any policies mutually agreed by the three consultants: a detailed exposition of this relationship was given in Chapter 5.

The pathology-complex in the same hospital group included the following staff:

– a consultant microbiologist (regarded as the 'chief' pathologist)

- a consultant histologist
- a consultant haematologist
- a clinical assistant in cytology
- a physicist
- a principal biochemist
- one senior chief technician
- three other chief technicians
- a number of technicians of various grades
- a small number of clerical staff.

The 'extant' pattern of organization was seen[5] broadly as a number of separate but linked hierarchies shown in Figure 6.3.

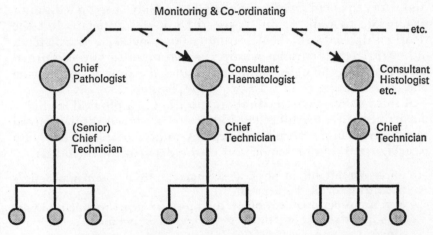

Figure 6.3   Organization of a Pathology-Complex

In contrast to the radiology department, each consultant had his own chief technician subordinate to him. The senior chief technician, who was a subordinate of the chief pathologist, had in addition to his special work in microbiology a cross-laboratory concern with general laboratory administration, supplies and training. For example, this senior chief technician provided a materials-supply service for the other chief technicians. However, he did not regard himself as in superior-subordinate relationship to the other

[5] This view was obtained in discussions with the chief pathologist, and his senior chief technician, and later confirmed by the local Project Steering Committee.

chief technicians. He also had special duties in the field of recruitment and training, and it was part of his job to arrange the allocation of technicians (most of whom were in training in various
stages), to various branches of the pathology-complex, according
to both service and training needs. At the time the senior chief
technician's role was diagnosed as simply service-giving. In retrospect one would probably want to add – and monitoring and co-
ordinating – although at the time of that particular project we were
not alive to the monitoring and co-ordinating concepts.

Thus at any one time each consultant (and for this analysis the
chief biochemist seemed to rate as a consultant, though the positions of the cytologist and physicist were not so clear) had not only
his own permanent chief technician, but a body of seconded junior
technicians as well. Again, at the time of the initial project the
relationship between the consultants was diagnosed as collateral,
although later discussions within the consultant group concerned
suggested that the chief pathologist had some limited monitoring
and co-ordinating role, as reported in Chapter 5.

A third study of paramedical organization in a physical medicine
department in a teaching hospital group produced similar agreed
formulations of a several-tier hierarchy under consultant direction
(see Figure 6.4). The senior staff of the department included:

- three consultants in physical medicine, one of whom was designated director of the department;
- a group superintendent physiotherapist, six superintendent physiotherapists and about thirty or forty physiotherapists (some part-
  time);
- a group head occupational therapist with some fifteen assistants
  of various grades.[6]

In this case, one consultant, the director, was seen as accountable
for the provision of all physiotherapy and occupational therapy
services to meet the prescribed requirements of medical staff of the
hospitals in the group, and all the physiotherapists and occupational therapists were seen as accountable to him.

All three consultants would have the right to prescribe treatment in respect of their own patients to be carried out by physio-

[6] Discussion were held, and a final formulation agreed, with the director
of physical medicine, the group superintendent physiotherapist, three superintendent physiotherapists, and the group head occupational therapist.

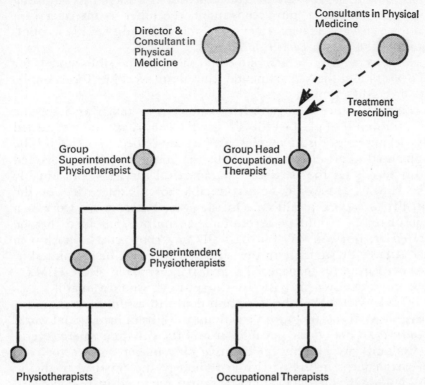

Figure 6.4   Organization of a Department of Physical Medicine

therapists and occupational therapists, as indeed would other consultants (for example, orthopaedic surgeons) in respect of theirs.

The Position of Consultants in Charge of Paramedical Departments

Having discovered these and other evidences of the considerable managerial roles of consultants in charge of paramedical departments, we were naturally led to question whether the position of such consultants was therefore necessarily different from that of their colleagues without paramedical staff. One possible distinction – that departmental consultants were all 'advisory', in contrast to their 'clinical' colleagues (see Chapter 5) – had to be abandoned in view of the existence of radiotherapists and directors of physical medicine, for example, with their own patients. We tried another line. Should the consultants concerned be considered to be filling two roles, one as a 'pure' consultant, the other as manager of a large service-giving department, and was the quality of his accountability different in each role?

More generally, in fact, one could see three possible models for the position of the 'departmental' consultant working, for example, in an H.M.C. group.

Firstly (Figure 6.5(a) – where radiology is taken as a specific illustration) it might be requisite for the consultant to be regarded as having two distinct roles as just described. He would be appointed to his managerial role by the hospital authority charged with supplying the particular paramedical service – presumably the H.M.C. He would be accountable to this authority for the quality of service produced. On the other hand, in his work as a consultant he would be accountable to no one provided that he stayed 'within bounds'; but basically in a contract-relationship to the R.H.B. Presumably in this situation he could be appointed or removed from his managerial role at the discretion of the H.M.C., but in either case his basic consultant-work would remain.

This model makes the large and doubtful assumption that it is possible to dissociate 'pure' consultant-work from managerial work. However, it does make possible sense of the situation where several consultants are eligible for the role of manager or director of a department, as in the particular radiology and physical medicine examples described above; and it is still regarded in project-work as a possible model for some situations.

Alternatively it might be that the consultant in charge should be regarded as accountable not to the H.M.C., but perhaps to the R.H.B., in his managerial role. The implication then is that it is the R.H.B., and not the H.M.C. that is accountable for the provision of X-ray services, or pathology services or whatever. However, this model (Figure 6.5(b)) does have the virtue of keeping only one source of contract-arrangements, only one employer, for the consultant concerned, in all aspects of his work. The H.M.C. might provide human and material resources and indeed monitor and co-ordinate the way they were used, but the accountability of the consultant in all situations would be only to the R.H.B.

But is it desirable that consultants should be in full managerial control of paramedical staff in such situations? A third alternative (Figure 6.5(c)) in principle at least, is that accountability for the

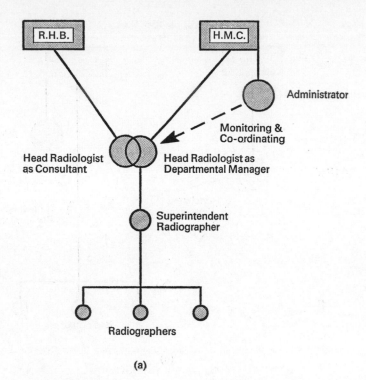

(a)

R.H.B.

H.M.C.

Administrator

Monitoring &
Co-ordinating

Head Radiologist
as Consultant

Head Radiologist as
Departmental Manager

Superintendent
Radiographer

Radiographers

R.H.B.

H.M.C.

Head
Radiologist

Administrator

Monitoring &
Co-ordinating

Superintendent
Radiographer

Radiographers

(b)

*Figure 6.5   Three Basic Alternatives for the Management of
Paramedical Work*

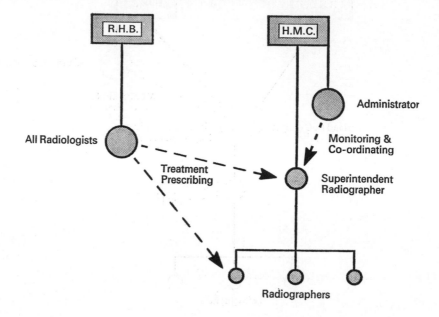

(c)
Figure 6.5 (continued)

management of each paramedical department might, above senior technician level, rest with some senior administrator, or even directly with the H.M.C. itself. The function of associated medical staff (pathologists, radiologists and so on) might then be:

(1) to prescribe specific treatment or investigations to be carried out for their own patients, or for investigations to be carried out so that they could provide reports and advice;
(2) to provide technical advice (directly or through medical committees) on how the department ought to be run or developed.

The resulting situation would put these medical staff in a relation to paramedical staff analogous to that, say, of surgeon or physician to nursing staff, a *treatment-prescribing* rather than a *superior-subordinate* relationship.[7]

[7] In the first and third cases there are of course two further sub-alternatives:
(1) That a senior administrator might play a monitoring and co-ordinating role in relation to the paramedical or medical head.
(2) That a senior administrator might be in superior-subordinate relationship to the head of the department.

So far, in project-discussion, we have not perceived a strong consensus for any one of these three basic possibilities. Most consultants with whom we have tested the ideas tend to view the third possibility as unworkable, and perhaps, to prefer the second; but many administrators on the other hand, defend the third. One argument posed is that doctors are not usually trained managers, and should therefore leave management to those who are (the administrators). The counter which neatly offsets it, is that of all eligible senior staff, only doctors in appropriate specialties are likely to appreciate the full range of problems, technical and others, of the paramedical staff concerned, and thus present themselves as 'natural' managers under whose control the paramedical staff may gravitate.

Of course, local factors may resolve the situation. Where for example there is no appointed director of physical medicine, then the physiotherapists and occupational therapists seem extantly *not* to gravitate to another consultant, but to stand on their own, or be regarded as subordinate to the local chief administrator. The same sometimes appears to happen to radiographers where there is only a part-time radiologist.

Other Organizational Positionings for Paramedical Staff

This then brings us back to the organizational position in general of paramedical staff. Where they do not naturally gravitate to the management of consultants (or where it is explicitly decided not to position them thus) which of the other two alternatives spelt out at the start of this chapter is appropriate, and for which classes of paramedical staff? To what extent can administrative staff of appropriate seniority be put *realistically* in a full managerial relationship to paramedical staff? And where paramedical staff are not subordinate to any consultants, do the latter nevertheless carry treatment-prescribing authority?

Leaving aside the groups of paramedical staff who (as we suggest) are extantly subordinate to consultants in most situations, we are now dealing then with the remainder of the list given at the start of the chapter, i.e.

> art therapists
> biochemists
> cardiological technicians

chiropodists
clinical psychologists
dietitians
medical artists
medical photographers
medical social workers
pharmacists
physicists
speech therapists

A few representatives of these various groups of staff with whom we have discussed their role have argued that they are indeed independent therapists, with their own patients, received by referral from consultants or general practitioners, and as such not eligible to be managed, or instructed on clinical matters by consultants or by anybody else. This position has been argued, for example, by a dietitian with whom we have worked, a chiropodist, a clinical psychologist, and a speech therapist.[8] One chief medical social worker with whom we have worked has seen herself as essentially independent of medical prescription. Another in a general hospital, and a psychiatric social worker in a psychiatric hospital saw the doctor, however, in a treatment-prescribing relationship. In any case one would hesitate to use the phrase 'independent therapist' of each and every social worker, as we have the considered and recorded the view of at least one chief medical social worker that other social workers in her department are subordinate to her, whilst there is evidence too from the local authority field that social workers are hierarchically-organized within their own discipline.[9]

On the other hand, whilst our explorations[10] have suggested that pharmacists too are hierarchically organized under chief pharmacists, there is little question that pharmacists are in fact subject to the treatment-prescribing (or perhaps service-seeking) authority of doctors. Pharmacists do and should query prescriptions for drugs where they feel that better or other alternatives are

[8] Whether consultants would generally agree with this view is not known. A recent D.H.S.S. circular (HM (71) 82) takes the bull by the horns in advocating that the dietitian should be responsible to the senior administrative officer of the Group or hospital in which she is employed.
[9] See Rowbottom and Hey (1970).
[10] With three chief pharmacists in different hospital groups.

possible, or where they feel that possible side-effects of prescribed drugs may have been overlooked; but in the end the doctor is seen as having the final word. A similar situation holds of course in nursing.

The final question to be considered, then, is whether those para-medical staff who are not independent therapists and not for one reason or other subordinate to any consultant, can be effectively managed by administrative staff. Should or could the chief pharma-cist or the head medical social worker, or the superintendent physiotherapist (in the absence of a director of physical medicine) be subordinate to an administrator of appropriate seniority (see Figure 6.6(b))? Or is each by virtue of a special profession ex-pertise, necessarily an independent officer of the employing author-ity, whose work can at most be co-ordinated and monitored by administrative staff (see Figure 6.6(a))?[11]

No clear answers to these questions have been suggested by the research so far.[12] As we suggested in Chapter 4, one necessary characteristic of a managerial (superior-subordinate) relationship is that the manager shall be able to comprehend, in full, the work

[11] Due note may be taken here of the Noel-Hall Report (1971) which although again chiefly about grading and career structures certainly gives also at least strong *indications* of possible new organization in pharmacy. Pharmacists and technicians would be 'working under the general direction of an Area Pharmacist' (Para. 4.35). Area Pharmacists would be 'responsible to the H.M.C., Board of Governors or Board of Management providing the service for the other authorities' (Para. 4.34). A Regional Pharmacist in an advisory capacity should be appointed (Para. 4.30), who might be a 'member of the staff of the Senior Administrative Medical Officers ... provided his right of access to the Board on pharmaceutical matters is preserved' (Para. 4.31). Perhaps this means that the S.A.M.O. would carry a monitoring and co-ordinating role.

[12] The question has been discussed with all the paramedical staff involved in field project-work, listed in an earlier footnote in this chapter. Leaving aside those who definitely saw themselves as accountable to a consultant it has been extremely difficult to reach any concensus of view on this question from the rest, or often enough, indeed, any clear view in individual cases. In preliminary discussion many of the people concerned, particularly the more junior in status would readily agree to being accountable (in some sense) to administration. (One respondent actually claimed that she was 'responsible to the office'!) However later and more analytical discussions have aften thrown doubt on the adequacy of these original formulations. It is possible that we (the researchers) do not yet understand the nature of this area well enough to be able to help those in it to reach formulations that really 'grip'.

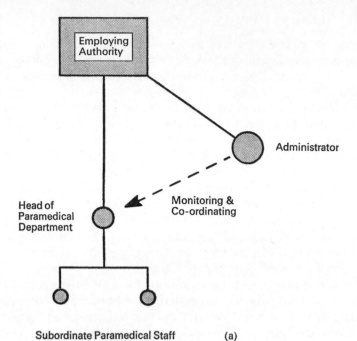

Employing
Authority

Administrator

Head of
Paramedical
Department

Monitoring &
Co-ordinating

Subordinate Paramedical Staff   (a)

Employing
Authority

Administrator

Head of Paramedical Department

Subordinate Paramedical Staff   (b)

*Figure 6.6   Alternative Positions for Paramedical Staff not Subordinate
to Consultants*

of the subordinate. If he is unable to do this, he cannot produce any satisfactory *total* assessment of the subordinate's performance. and of course, he will not feel happy to be held accountable for the totality of the subordinate's work.

Few administrators would claim that they could perform the work of pharmacists, or physiotherapists, or medical social workers, but the issue is not of ability to do the work of one's subordinates. The question is: may administrators of appropriate capacity reasonably be expected to be able to *comprehend* this work? Could they be expected to deal effectively not only with 'administrative' problems raised by the paramedical staff concerned, but with 'technical' problems as well?[13] If the answer is no, then it is likely that the relationship can be no stronger than monitoring and co-ordinating. In this case, the main thread of accountability would proceed directly from the head of each paramedical department to the governing body, and the assumption would then be that this head would have some right of direct access to that governing body.

Conclusion

To summarize, our research to date has strongly suggested that certain classes of paramedical staff – notably, laboratory technicians, radiographers, physiotherapists and occupational therapists – are requisitely organized in hierarchies headed by medical consultants. Although there are several views of the requisite position of such consultants, it is perhaps the case that their position is no different in essentials from that of any other consultants. All consultants have certain material and human resources under their direct control which, provided they stay within certain well-established bounds of contract law and professional practice, they may deploy as they think best. These particular consultants have relatively large numbers of human resources to help them, in the shape of paramedical staff, but perhaps are no more subject to authoritative direction in respect of the services they produce than any other consultant.

On the other hand certain other categories of paramedical staff

[13] This of course comes back to the question of the core-knowledge of a profession, and the extent to which it is or is not susceptible to grasp by the layman – the issue discussed in relation to doctors in Chapter 5. Here we are talking – in Etzioni's terms – of the 'semi-professions' (Etzioni 1969)

– notably social workers, pharmacists, and numbers of rarer specialties – are not normally subordinate to consultants, though they may
or may not be subject (in contrast) to their direction on treatment
or services required. Whether these latter categories of paramedical
workers can be made subordinate to administrators of appropriate
capacity, or whether by the nature of their professional expertise
this is unrealistic, is as yet an unresolved question.

7 Organization of Nursing Staff

At the time of writing the scope of our project-work in the field of nursing, at least in terms of numbers of nurses collaborating in project-work[1] has exceeded that in any other field.

In nursing, also, we have been working in a field of active organizational change, as on the one hand restyled nursing administration has gradually spread following the recommendations of the Salmon Report (1966), and on the other many non-nursing duties are gradually being given over to ward housekeeping teams following the recommendations of the Farrer Report (1968).

The half-dozen or so main groups of problems that we have repeatedly unearthed in project-work (as well as in conference-discussion) are shown below. Some stem from these temporary upheavals. Others are of more ancient origin. (Throughout we refer to 'wards' as a shorthand for all the areas where practical nursing is carried out, including therefore theatres and clinics.)

(1) What is the real role of the nurse on the ward? How is it that even as 'non-nursing' duties are (apparently) removed from nurses, they still retain this feeling of being jack of all trades, of being the ones who cope with the residual problems that do not fall into anybody else's job?

(2) What are the exact relationships of nursing staff at ward level to the many other people whose work bears directly on the ward

[1] Up to the autumn of 1971 we have carried out field-projects in two teaching groups and five H.M.C. groups covering intensive individual discussions with about sixty nurses at ward or department level, about eighty nurses in administrative posts above ward level, and about forty nurses in teaching posts. In addition we have tested many of the emerging formulations in conferences with senior nurses from eighteen other H.M.C. groups from the N.W. Metropolitan Region.

or the patient: to housekeepers (where ward housekeeping schemes exist), cleaners, porters, linen-suppliers, physiotherapists, occupational therapists, dietitians and so on; and what authority (if any) do nurses carry in these relationships?

(3) The doctor is a key figure at ward level. Where does his authority begin and end, and how does it accord with the authority to organize nursing which rests within nursing administration?

(4) What is the best structure for the management of nursing? Is there to be one nurse firmly in charge of one ward, day or night, whether on duty or off? What is the best structure above ward-level? With the introduction of standardized 'Salmon' grades for nursing administrators, should it be assumed that the organizational relationships between any two nurses in consecutive grades is the same (Grade 10 to Grade 9, Grade 9 to 8 and so on)? How do all these new grades relate to doctors, and to the various levels of administration?

(5) What is the optimum relationship of nurse training to service nursing? Should one take precedence over the other? Who is to decide where trainee nurses are allocated or reallocated to work in various wards and departments?

(6) Are nurses in charge of small, geographically-remote hospitals (e.g. cottage hospitals) in a special position which requires a special definition of organizational relationships?

These problems are not 'academic'. We have found as great anxieties amongst nurses, particularly senior nurses, about their proper roles and organizational relationships as amongst any staff: newly-created Principal and Senior Nursing Officers fearful lest their attempts to establish direct contact with their wards and patients is seen as 'inability to delegate'; ex-matrons of small hospitals anxious lest group administration should more and more destroy their former independence; ward sisters trying with difficulty to accommodate to radical reorganization of ward-work demanded by doctors; tutors incensed to find that their trainees have to be switched once again, without consultation, to reinforce failing points in an overstretched nursing service.

In modern general hospitals, nurses find themselves at the very hub of a large and highly complex organization, and by and large, their training has left them blind to the real nature and adequacy of this organization and the elements of which it is composed.

The Real Role of the Nurse at Ward Level

The most immediate image of the work of the nurse on the ward shows her busy administering basic nursing care, medicines, and other prescribed treatment to the individual patient. Whilst it has not been part of our project-work at any point to produce an exhaustive and detailed list of all the activities undertaken by nurses on wards, a general view of the work of more senior ward nurses has gradually emerged from discussions which includes the following elements:

(1) administering basic nursing care to patients in need – attending to their cleanliness, feeding, and general bodily and mental comfort;

(2) administering specific treatment to patients in response to medical prescriptions, or carrying out specific services in connection with treatment such as, for example, arranging for laboratory investigations, physiotherapy, or X-rays;

(3) ensuring that all other activities which bear on the patient happen as they should, and in an orderly fashion – admission and discharge, contact with relatives, visits from social workers; chiropodists, voluntary workers, barbers, etc.;

(4) ensuring the general cleanliness, order, and safety, of the ward, through such things as monitoring the quality of cleaning work done, requisitioning maintenance for buildings and equipment which fall into disrepair, and ensuring that the visiting of patients is carried out in an orderly manner;

(5) ensuring that trainee nurses of various kinds allocated to the ward are given a due variety of practical experience and training. (See note at end of chapter.)

In short, nurses play not only a special role in a therapeutic team alongside other members of that team – the doctors, the social workers, the physiotherapists, and so on – but over and above this they act as what might be called *local site managers*, in ensuring that all the services which flow to a particular patient in a particular site (the ward) are continuously available and well co-ordinated.

It falls to nurses, and to no other hospital staff, to monitor the needs and problems of the patient day and night – to cope with clinical emergencies as best they can whilst calling for medical help, to delay admissions, to hasten discharges, to cope in the last resort with failures in cleaning, breakdowns in catering, shortages in linen, and so on. In spite of the fact that many duties not requiring nursing skills but formerly carried out by nurses, have now been transferred to auxiliaries, cleaners, housekeepers, clerks and the like, it is still the job, at least of senior nursing staff on the wards, to monitor and co-ordinate (if not positively to manage) the work of these people.

Relationship of Ward Nursing Staff to Paramedical and Supporting Staff

This naturally leads on to the question of the exact nature of the organizational relationships of senior ward staff to paramedical and other staff whose work bears closely on the work of the ward.

At an earlier stage in the research we tended to categorize all these relationships, perhaps too readily, as either collateral or service-giving (see Chapter 4). True, a number of departments do appear to be in a straightforward service-giving relationship to nurses on the wards – for example, pharmacy, laundry and linen stores, (general) supplies, central sterile supplies departments, engineering, and building. Even so, supplies departments sometimes seemed to have a more positive role than merely service-giving. They appear on occasion to be vetting the judgement of nurses, where major items were claimed to be needed; whereas a straightforward service-relationship would suggest that the supplies department, over and above advising on suitable sources of purchase, should have no more authority than that of monitoring adherence to budget limits or standardized sources of supply where firm policies existed on these.

Cleaning staff, though on the face of it in straightforward service-giving relationship to nursing staff, have not in fact been quite in this relationship in some general hospitals where we have studied the situation. In these particular cases, the work of cleaners, organized under a separate domestic department, was clearly determined by a programme specifically agreed between senior domestic staff and senior nursing staff. Thus it was deliberately arranged that the ward nursing staff did not have discretion to decide what cleaning work was or was not required as they saw fit, though they might always, of course, raise questions of the need for change of programme with the more senior nurses who negotiated it. However, ward staff were certainly still to be concerned with cleanliness. This concern should be expressed through a monitoring relationship, in which the senior ward nursing staff checked on the results of the cleaning work done, remonstrated if need be with the cleaners themselves, and if getting no satisfaction there raised the matter as a complaint with the local domestic supervisor. (The organization of cleaning and housekeeping staff is discussed in more detail in the next chapter.)

Relationships with catering staff again turned out to be complex. On the face of things, again, the relationship was a straightforward service-giving one. But were catering staff, in preparing food for patients, giving a service to the nursing staff, or to patients themselves? Catering managers, for example, reported that they sometimes visited the wards themselves to check with patients (not just with nursing staff) how well the food was liked. These considerations suggest that the relationship between catering and nursing staff is a collateral one rather than a service-giving one, though once again nurses had also to monitor and co-ordinate the work of the catering department to some extent, in checking for themselves, for example, the quality or temperature of food received, or in progressing or delaying the supply of food and serving of meals in order to co-ordinate these with other activities on the ward.

Relationships with physiotherapists, occupational therapists, and other paramedical staff who visit the ward, raise further organizational points. Both paramedical staff and nurses are separately concerned with the treatment and care of patients. On the surface their relationship appears to be collateral. The provisos are twofold. Firstly, collateral relationships, as discussed in Chapter 4, imply the presence of an authoritative cross-over point in any matter of dispute. Given, for example, the normal organizational placing of physiotherapists under a consultant, it is difficult to see a cross-over point with authority to set policies binding both on nurses and on physiotherapists. Secondly, as we have indicated, nurses have a duty to monitor the provision of physiotherapy and co-ordinate it with other provision for the patient in a way which is not reciprocated by the physiotherapist in relation to provision of nursing care.

Where ward housekeeping schemes have been or are being instituted, ward housekeepers are in the classical 'dual-influence' organization described in Chapter 4. In consequence, any of the four types of situation described might in theory apply – outposted service-giving, attachment, functional monitoring, and co-ordinating or secondment. These possibilities are again explored in more detail in the following chapter.

The real issues here are of course not simply what organizational labels to put on these relationships, but (what always lies underneath the labelling activity) issues of appropriate behaviour, relationship and response. Who exactly is accountable for doing what? Whose job is it to check the quality of food, of cleaning? Whose job is it to deal with complaints about poor food or lack of cleanliness? Whose job is it to programme the supply of food and carrying out of cleaning programmes?

Even where straightforward service-relationships prevail, as in certain of the cases described above, a specific problem arises in many hospitals of the kind identified in this extract from a report of a project in a large teaching hospital.

A major problem experienced by nursing staff lay in the relationship with services. Ward sisters often found difficulty in obtaining adequate services such as cleaning, linen, porterage and supplies. Ward sisters could not turn to anyone clearly felt to be in the appropriate position to deal with the problem, once a direct approach to the service-givers had been made. Such matters were therefore dealt with by referral to senior nurses or to the administrative staff in control of the service-giving department. These referrals did not succeed in clearing up the problem since the nursing side was organized separately from the administrative and service side. The Chief Nursing Officer could not instruct a ward cleaner, nor could the House Governor instruct a ward sister. Decisions binding on both sides could be taken nowhere below the level of the Board of Governors. The day-to-day problems arising on the services side could not therefore be properly resolved.

Here then is a situation in which the cross-over point is so far removed organizationally from the point of day-to-day interaction that resolution of unresolved problems becomes virtually impossible. Here, nurses having lost the burden of responsibility for providing certain services themselves, find that they have also lost, perhaps to an intolerable degree, the right of control that accompanied that burden.

Relationship of Nurses to Doctors

Who manages nurses: doctors or other nurses? The practically universal finding from our research is that the real managerial link is from nurse to nurse, not from doctor to nurse. It is senior nurses who are accountable for the provision of nursing services, who select and train junior nursing staff, assign them to particular positions, assess them, and if need be initiate transfer or dismissal.

Nurses are not subordinate to doctors, but they are of course subject to their instructions on the treatment or services to be carried out in respect of individual patients. (The precise role of the doctors in this situation has been discussed in Chapter 5.) This *treatment-prescribing* authority spans all the work of nursing, though certain parts of nursing might appear at first sight perhaps to fall outside it. We had suspected, for example, at an early stage in the research that midwives might be in a different position, in that, given the nature of their work, they sometimes find themselves 'treating' patients in the absence of medical prescription. However it is clearly acknowledged that where a doctor is brought into the situation (and it is a midwife's responsibility to do so when the need for medical care becomes evident) the midwife has become as subject to medical prescription as any other nurse.[2]

Again, at an early stage in the research we surmised that there was perhaps an area of nursing – the 'basic' nursing activity described above – in which nurses practised autonomously and independently of doctors; but again, on exploration and discussion this turned out to be an inadequate view. Although it is true that doctors do not usually make prescriptions about basic nursing care – washing, feeding, linen-changing and so on, for sick patients – it is clear that they have a right to do so which is exercised usually only in situations where commonplace nursing practices are *not* to be applied for some clinical reason or other.

Of course this does not mean that doctors may prescribe what treatment they like, without any limit. One set of limits arises out of what is legal or ethical. Obviously no nurse should administer a known poison in lethal dose to a patient, however firm the prescription. Many nurses, on grounds of religious belief, will not engage in abortions in certain circumstances. More important per-

[2] The Central Midwives' Board Handbook (1962) states:
'If a midwife is acting in a case in which a registered medical practitioner is also engaged she must carry out such instructions concerning the care of the patient and the infant as may be given to her by the practitioner subject to compliance with the rules of the Board.'

haps, discussions with many nurses have suggested a distinction between questions of treatment of the *individual* patient, in which the doctor does carry ultimate and unilateral authority, and questions of *general* procedures or organization of treatment, in which mutual agreement is necessary (see Chapter 5).

A third field in which some doubt has been cast on the treatment-prescribing authority of the doctor is that of psychiatric nursing. Several psychiatrists in discussing this question have been loath to acknowledge a unilateral right to prescribe treatment. They argue that in psychiatric practice (a) the nurse is often better able to judge the appropriate 'social' treatment for particular patients as they are in far more regular contact with the patients than the doctor is, and see more of their general behaviour and responses, and (b) it might be difficult or impossible to prescribe comprehensively the behaviour required of a psychiatric nurse in what is, after all, a 'total therapeutic' situation. These arguments would presumably apply with greatest strength in an explicit, therapeutic community approach.

We have not so far pursued this last discussion to any definite conclusion, but the following questions appear to be relevant:

(a) does the psychiatrist carry treatment-prescribing authority in relation to physical treatment (by drugs, electrotherapy, etc.)?

(b) would the psychiatrist consider that he had at least negative authority of veto in relation to any treatment, social or physical, which he considered dangerous or not in the best interests of the patient?

In the end one returns to what is possibly the fundamental criterion for deciding whether or not the consultant should possess clinical autonomy – that discussed in Chapter 5. Does the patient entrust himself to the care of one identified psychiatrist, and does he expect that psychiatrist to take total charge of his treatment? If so, treatment-prescribing authority seems unavoidable. If not, if, for example, the patient is entrusting his case to an agency, or to some sort of 'community', then treatment-prescribing authority may no longer be a necessity.

These special cases apart, the position of the ward-nurse vis-à-vis doctors and more senior nurses does generally seem to be as shown in Figure 7.1. Nurses at all levels are part of one managerial hierarchy (see Chapter 4). Doctors give treatment-prescriptions to ward

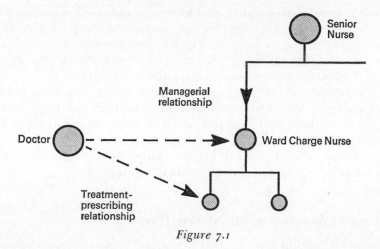

Figure 7.1

charge nurses (or other senior nurses on wards), who either carry them out themselves, or ensure that other nurses, junior nurses, or nurses on the shifts, do so.[3]

It may be, of course, that special situations arise where nursing staff are seconded to the direct management of doctors, but we have come across surprisingly few examples in our fieldwork. Two possible cases have been firstly, the case of a nurse working full-time in an X-ray department, and secondly a nurse working full-time in a venereology clinic. Might there also be cases of nurses working in highly-specialized or experimental areas who are in effect seconded for various periods of time to work under the doctor concerned?

This in fact raises a more general doubt, which has been expressed to us by at least one senior nurse in the project. As various areas of nursing become more specialized – theatre work, intensive-

[3] The Salmon Report (1966) refers to the ward sister as being under the *control* of the Matron (structural authority) but in matters of medical treatment acting in accordance with the *directions* of the medical staff (sapiental authority) (Para. 4.1.). As defined in that Report 'structural authority' obviously corresponds to what we here call 'managerial' or 'superior-subordinate' authority (See Appendix A). But we have found no one concept to equate to 'sapiental' authority (Appendix 1, Salmon Report); in fact, as indicated in Chapter 4 we have found the need to define many different kinds of authority other than managerial in order to describe the variety of relationships extant, and presumably necessary, in hospital organization.

care work, renal-dialysis work and so on – it may be impossible for senior nursing administrators to have sufficient grasp of the full-range of specialties to become capable of assessing the work of nurses in every specialty. If so, the simple nursing hierarchy of successive superior-subordinate relationships disappears, and a more complex organizational form comes into being, in which the superior-subordinate links stop at some point (or perhaps carry through to medical staff) leaving senior nursing administrators in something less than full managerial relationships.

Nevertheless this doubt lies on the margins of the research and is far from being well-tested or generally accepted.

The Detailed Structure of the Nursing Hierarchy

The general assumption in this research so far, an assumption which has received widespread acceptance, is that the basic structure of nursing organization is that of a pure hierarchy. Put in another way, the assumption is that the most senior nurse in the situation (sometimes that of a hospital, sometimes that of the Group) is accountable for the work of all nurses in the situation, and has, or should have, full managerial authority in relation to them – the right to select, prescribe work, assess, and transfer or dismiss.

Given this basic structure, the question is – and it is one of the most important questions facing the nursing profession at the moment – *exactly* what sort of managerial structure is needed within the basic hierarchy, for the most efficient organization of nursing work?

In order to appreciate the full significance of this question it is necessary for a moment to step aside from the description of the research analysis and findings to consider the general situation of nursing as the recommendations of the Salmon Report are gradually introduced.

Prior to the Report, there were three main categories of senior nursing staff:

(1) ward sisters or charge nurses, as their names imply, in charge of wards;
(2) matrons, in charge of hospitals; and
(3) a variety of nurses variously called deputy matrons, assistant

matrons, administrative sisters, etc., poised organizationally somewhere between the two.

The title 'matron' was used of posts with the widest variety of responsibility, from that of the nurse in charge of a cottage hospital of, say, thirty beds, to that of the nurse in charge of a large teaching hospital of, say, eight hundred beds.

One of the main recommendations of the Salmon Report was the establishment of a system of uniform gradings for all nursing staff, ranging from staff-nurse (Grade 5) to the chief nurse in charge of a sizeable group of hospitals (Grade 10). In implementing these proposals each of the grades has tended in practice to be associated with a particular title,[4] as follows:

Grade 10 – chief nursing officer (C.N.O.)
Grade 9 – principal nursing officer (P.N.O.)
Grade 8 – senior nursing officer (S.N.O.)
Grade 7 – nursing officer (N.O.)
Grade 6 – charge nurse
Grade 5 – staff nurse, or equivalent

So much for the grading system, but what about the nature of the executive relationships? It has been our uniform experience in the research, in working in field-projects with nurses in six Hospital Groups where Salmon schemes were in process of implementation, that a certain assumption tends to be adopted consciously or unconsciously. The assumption is that every step in Salmon grade marks a uniform organizational relationship, close if not identical to a managerial relationship. Actually even this is not quite the truth of the matter. The truth is that there is often no clear dis-

---

[4] The Salmon Report did not suggest that uniform titles be adopted, but did frown on the use of titles such as 'assistant' and 'deputy', and there has been a tendency to avoid these. In fact the use of the standardized titles described above in the text (which are actually no more or less meaningful than assistant or deputy), each associated with one particular grade has led, unintentionally, to a very difficult situation. It has now become difficult to ask the quite legitimate question 'What is the correct grade for this post?'. Since the post in question has probably already been entitled 'nursing officer' or 'principal nursing officer' or whatever, the grading appears to be automatic. What is needed is a vocabulary of titles for posts which are quite separate from grades, and in fact the association of all the obvious kinds of titles with specific grades is not only unnecessary, but has created a situation of shortage of possible non-grade-attached titles!

tinction at all made between grading concepts and concepts of organizational relationships.[5]

The Confusion of Ranking and Grading

Strictly speaking, a 'grade' in the context of organizational employment, is nothing more nor less than an arbitrarily-created zone in a continuous salary scale. The Salmon Committee recommended five grades: they were equally at liberty to recommend ten or twenty had so many been convenient.[6]

'Grade' may be contrasted with quite a different concept, that of 'rank', which can be defined as the level in a managerial hierarchy. In this concept, a difference of one rank thus corresponds to a superior-subordinate step in executive relationships within a hierarchy. (Note that the concept applies only within hierarchical organizations – see Chapter 4.)

It will therefore be purely fortuitous in any organization if a jump of one grade corresponds to a jump of one rank in the requisite organization-structure. For whereas the number of grades in a grading structure can be expanded or contracted more or less at will, without great inconvenience, it is probably the case that numbers of managerial levels in organizations of given size cannot.[7]

---

[5] In fact, as things go at the moment it is easily possible to confuse three different sorts of language, that of *organizational relationship*, that of *grade* and (as previously noted) that of *post title*. Thus the title 'senior nursing officer' means automatically 'Grade 8' and may be taken unthinkingly to imply invariably a superior-subordinate relationship with any nurses in Grade 7 in the same part of the organization.

[6] In fact it later turned out to be convenient to subdivide most Salmon Grades into three 'steps'.

[7] Common sense alone would support the idea that there could be too many or too few managerial levels for a given size of organization. Jaques (Brown and Jaques, 1965) has advanced an important theoretical analysis of this idea. Drawing on the one hand an empirical evidence of the relationships between levels of work (as measured by time-span of discretion) and felt superior-subordinate relationships, and on the other, on speculation as to the necessary difference in individual 'capacity' between a superior and his subordinate for optimum working of the managerial relationship, he has posed a precise hypothesis of the optimum number of managerial levels – up to six for the largest hierarchies – for any given size of organization measured in terms of the level of work implied for the chief executive.

It was found in the Glacier Metal Company (Brown, 1965), where much of the research was carried out on which this theory was based, that four

In fact, we have found much evidence to suggest that if the assumption is made that every step in Salmon Grade in nursing corresponds to a step in executive rank, this will be wrong. In particular, in discussion with nurses in the middle zones, we have found frequent uncertainty in ward-areas as to whether the S.N.O.s and N.O.s, either or both, could play full-managerial roles. In 'departments' – theatres, outpatients, accident and emergency, and in small hospitals – we have found doubts expressed as to whether the nurses at the charge-nurse level could play full managerial roles.

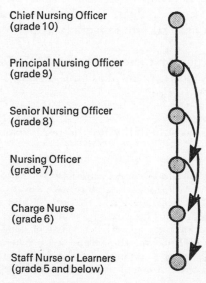

Chief Nursing Officer
(grade 10)

Principal Nursing Officer
(grade 9)

Senior Nursing Officer
(grade 8)

Nursing Officer
(grade 7)

Charge Nurse
(grade 6)

Staff Nurse or Learners
(grade 5 and below)

Figure 7.2   Apparent Five-rank Structures in Nursing
(with frequent by-passing)

This doubt is often expressed in the form of anxiety about by-passing. Nurses, apparently at levels once-removed, are seen to be 'interfering' in areas which should be being managed by nurses at the intermediate level. The senior nurses, in separate discussions, sometimes reveal their conflict between 'delegating as good managers should' (on the one hand) and 'keeping in touch with

management levels only were needed at that particular stage of the Company's development. However, it was found convenient to have a grading system which had *three times* as many levels, i.e. three grades per rank.

the work of the wards', as their intuition leads them to see desirable, on the other.[8]

Managerial, Supervisory, and Staff, Roles in Nursing

Once again, we see a familiar picture. A group of people, conscious of some general organizational scheme which they suppose they are to follow, at the same time unconsciously adapting the scheme as they go, to fit the total reality of their work situation as they find it. In helping nurses to become more aware of their organizational position, and of the range of possibilities open to them, we have drawn their attention to at least two important alternatives[9] to straightforward managerial roles, namely supervisory roles, and staff-officer roles.

The general nature of these roles has been fully defined in Chapter 4, but it is worth re-emphasizing certain features in relation to nursing organization.

Full-managerial roles
– carry continuing accountability for the performance, training and

[8] The complementary doubt of course, expressed by many nurses in middle or lower positions is just who is the real 'boss'. As Revans says 'a hospital is an institution cradled in anxiety ... In situations of anxiety one seeks two supports: a senior on whom one can rely, and an understanding of what happens next' (Revans 1964, p. 64). His work has of course been primarily concerned with ways of fulfilling the second requirement through better communication and learning processes, but the anxiety that also arises in the absence of the first requirement is real and important enough in its own right.

[9] The Salmon Report itself did not of course assume that the organizational relationships between nurses in any two adjacent grades would be the same. They distinguished between *full control* – the juniors being responsible to the superior – and *actual control*, the juniors being responsible to a nurse in the level next above her but reporting to the immediate superior (Para. 1.10). This is probably close to our distinction between managerial and supervisory relationships. At the same time, the Report refers (Para. 1.5) to three levels of management – top management (Grades 9 and 10) who decide policy, middle management (Grades 8 and 7) who programme policy, and first-line management (Grades 6 and 5), those who execute policy. These levels do not however, necessarily correspond to 'ranks' as defined above, and generally the distinction between policy-making, programming, and execution does not appear to have been of great practical use in implementation.

development of junior staff over relatively long periods of time (i.e. many weeks or months);
- in consequence, are the natural points for making the assessments of staff that count, and have weight;
- carry continuing accountability for the development of procedures and organization;
- cannot be (regularly) by-passed without undermining their position.

Supervisory Roles
- carry 'shift-accountability' only for staff and procedures;
- contribute to, but do not make, final assessments of staff;
- can be by-passed as required by managerial roles, and must be by-passed from time-to-time if the accountable nursing manager is to have direct contact with all her subordinates;
- frequently 'act-up' for the higher managerial role to cover absence.

Staff-Officer Roles
- do not carry direct accountability for the provision of nursing services, though their occupants may from time-to-time, in a different role, deputize for other nurses with managerial or supervisory roles;
- are concerned with helping to formulate policies (e.g. for recruitment and training); and, given approved policies, with preparing and issuing detailed plans for implementation.

Supervisory Roles in Nursing

Perhaps the most obvious example of the use of supervisory roles in nursing arises at ward level. Where a staff-nurse or a senior trainee nurse is in charge for a shift, what is expected of them fits the supervisory pattern described above much better than it fits the managerial definition. (Here the managerial role is probably carried by the charge-nurse – but see later discussion.)

We have found supervisory roles at slightly higher levels in, for example, an outpatient clinic and in a theatre suite. In both these cases, nurses of Charge Nurse Grade were put in charge of teams of more junior nurses for the course of particular clinic or theatre sessions, but the membership of teams changed from session to session. In each of these situations the N.O. in charge of the department was seen as the real 'boss', and the charge-nurse in a temporary supervisory position.

At a higher level still, the outcome of a project in a maternity division[10] suggested recognition of the need for supervisory, rather than managerial, roles of S.N.O. and N.O. grade as shown in Figure 7.3(b) (senior night staff and tutorial staff are not shown). The charts drawn up in the initial stages of Salmon implementations showed an organization as in Figure 7.3(a). In fact, discussions with the senior nurses suggested:

(a) that the head of the division needed and was able to keep in direct touch with the heads of the various wards and other units;
(b) but that she could not single-handedly manage the work of these units all day long, seven days a week, and that high-level supervisors were needed to help support the nurses at ward and unit level, some of whom might be relatively inexperienced at their jobs;
(c) that it would be more helpful for these high-level supervisors to cover the full range of activities than for each to specialize, in view of the duty-pattern; but that when each were on duty together a rough working division of supervision by area would be employed;
(d) that whilst the N.O.s would act as supervisors to charge-nurses, the S.N.O. would in turn, act as a supervisor to the N.O.s where supervision was needed – i.e. there would be a hierarchy of supervision.

Staff-Officer Roles in Nursing

A common example of a staff-officer role in nursing is that often carried under the title 'allocation officer' (see Figure 7.4). We have explored such roles fully in at least three Groups and found that the essential staff-officer nature of the role, once suggested, has rapidly been recognized by the occupants of the role and most other senior nursing staff concerned.

The main functions in these roles are usually:

(1) allocation of learner nurses to wards and departments, in accordance with the demands of service and training programmes;
(2) arrangement of induction and post-registration training courses;
(3) recruitment;
(4) maintenance of personnel records.

[10] Involving the P.N.O. in charge, an S.N.O., two N.O.s, and three Charge Nurses, and later, the C.N.O. of the Group.

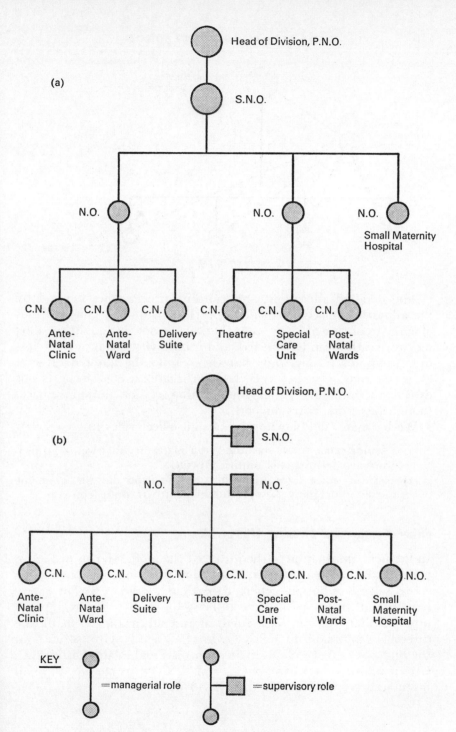

Figure 7.3 Organization of a Maternity Division (a) *Manifest Organization and* (b) *Requisite Organization*

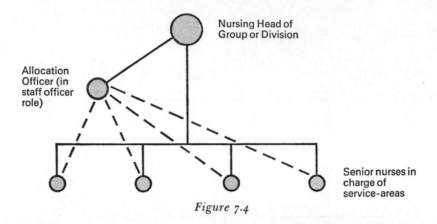

Figure 7.4

The detailed allocations and training programmes devised by the allocations officer, provided they lie within the general lines of agreed policies, are seen as authoritative, not just advisory. This means that they can be queried, and if necessary taken to the crossover point for testing, but that they cannot be ignored at will, as advice may. On the other hand, the allocations officer is not directly accountable either for training or for nursing-service, though her work bears on both.

We have also found examples of staff officer roles in:

(1) a senior nurse tutor, seconded to a maternity division, who programmed training for pupil midwives;
(2) a senior nurse tutor in a theatre suite who did the same for nurses undergoing post-graduate theatre training courses.

Other Features of Nursing Hierarchies

In further confirmation of the idea that the model shown in Figure 7.2 is far from descriptive of all nursing situations, we have come across several situations where a particular grade was not represented at all in one part of the nursing hierarchy – for example, a proposal that N.O.s in some medical and surgical areas should be directly accountable to a P.N.O. in one H.M.C. Group, without the interposition of S.N.O.s in any capacity; and in another H.M.C. Group a situation where N.O.s and S.N.O.s in charge of small hospitals were accountable directly to the C.N.O.

We have also come across an example of successive grades, apparently working in collateral relationships, the people concerned being senior tutors (S.N.O.s) and tutors (N.O.s) in a large school of nursing. Manifestly, the tutors were accountable to the senior tutors for their work, but in fact saw themselves as accountable directly to the principal tutor (P.N.O.).

'Natural' Managerial Roles

Is it possible to chart generally where full-managerial roles might be predicted to arise in nursing? Perhaps some help may be gained by looking for what might be called the 'natural' managerial units. By this we mean, broadly, some unit that has an obvious identity of its own apart from lines drawn on some organization chart; a unit that has obvious boundaries defined perhaps geographically, or in terms of special function, or special clientele.

Possible examples of 'natural' managerial units from a nursing point of view are:

- a hospital group as a whole;
- any individual hospital so geographically remote as to require its own self-contained organization;
- a school of nursing;
- a maternity division;
- a theatre suite;
- an accident and emergency department;
- an outpatients department.

We have found little doubt in the area covered by this research, that the nurses in charge of such units are regarded as carrying full-managerial roles, whatever their grade – and the grades encountered here include examples of all from N.O. upward.

What about the ward itself? Is this a 'natural' managerial unit? Traditionally, it has been, and the ward sister has been regarded as in 'full control' of her ward whether or not she was temporarily absent (Salmon, Para. 4.13). In the research, we have come across isolated examples of charge-nurses in ward-situations where another, 'second' or 'junior', charge nurse was also employed on the ward, who expressed some doubt as to the reality of their full-managerial role. But the strong consensus of view encountered in the research is that there certainly ought to be one nurse in clear

managerial control of the ward and of all nursing staff on the ward
– at least, all the nursing staff on day duty.

In the end, of course, it all depends on how a 'ward' is defined.
As physical patterns of hospital layout, and patterns of care for
patients, change and evolve, it may be necessary to recognize new
'basic units' of nursing management, with a consequent need for
the redefinition of the associated managerial role.

Another possible advantage of distinguishing the real managerial
roles in nursing might be to allow a clearer definition of the important 'sideways' links between nurses and doctors, and nurses
and administrators. In the past, for example, doctors have tended
to see important links with nurses at two levels – ward sisters and
matrons. Now they are sometimes in situations where they are encouraged to think of making contacts with anything up to five
levels of nursing management, from Charge Nurse to C.N.O.[11]

We may speculate that if in a particular part of nursing organization full-managerial levels were established at say N.O. in charge
of a department, and P.N.O. in charge of a large division, then
these two levels would be the normal points of contact for doctors,
although on occasion they might find that in the absence of the
P.N.O. they were dealt with by her S.N.O. 'assistants', or in the
absence of the N.O. by her charge-nurse 'assistants'. The same
sorts of consideration would no doubt apply to contacts with
administrators, or members of other departments.

Continuing Need for Supervisory Roles

However, even having established the location of the 'natural'
managerial units and roles, there are other characteristics of nursing work which have gradually become clear to us as the study has
progressed, which all seem to point to the same and very specific
conclusion. Consider these facts for the moment.

(1) Nursing is a twenty-four-hour, seven-days-a-week service.
(2) Clinical or other problems, some with a high degree of urgency,
and requiring high-level skills to deal with them, can arise at
any time of the day or night.
(3) Owing to the heavy reliance on the use of nurses at various stages

[11] Again, the reaction of doctors to this new situation is legion. Many with
whom we have worked have seen 'Salmon' as the introduction of new hordes
of nursing administrators, adding nothing but confusion to the situation.

in a process of learning in the provision of a nursing service, the actual nursing skills available in any situation are very variable, and likely to need considerable reinforcement when in difficulties.

Unless managers are going to work around the clock, seven days a week, it is obvious that they will need support in managing the work of their subordinates – not just specialist staff support in the form of detailed planning (though this will indeed be needed in certain places) but more general, operational support in helping with emergencies, checking on work done, guiding, inducting, giving on-the-spot training, and so on. In other words (we reach the same general conclusion again) they need *supervisors* in considerable strength.

These facts and their implications are of course well understood (not necessarily in these terms) by nurses. One of the remarkable features of existing nursing organization is the highly developed and flexible way in which it is ensured that there shall always be someone clearly 'in charge' at various levels from the ward upwards. Senior nurses 'act-up', 'act-down', 'act-across', 'stand-in', and carry-out any number of similar organizational contortions in order to provide the necessary spread of supervisory skill. In all this the general rule is well understood, that higher grade is always in supervisory role to lower.

In a sense the problems of nursing organization are not those of inability to provide effective supervision, shift by shift. The problems are (contrary to the way our discussion has proceeded) in selecting out of the shifting complex of supervisory roles, the ones which are truly managerial. Which are the senior nurses who are expected to be working, not just from shift to shift, but over longer periods of time in developing staff, systems, and procedures; the proprietors, so-to-speak, of their own particular units?

Night Organization

Organization for night work raises again the general question of the nature of accountability of the ward charge nurse. Is she accountable for the work of all staff on the ward, day or night? Or are ward staff on night duty accountable directly to senior nursing staff themselves on night duty? The two possibilities can be stated more formally as follows:

First Possibility
Junior nursing staff on night duty are ultimately accountable to the
(day) head of the particular ward or unit in which they work. This
managerial role carries the long-term accountability for these night
staff, and for their methods of work. The senior night staff are there
to give immediate support, guidance and control, but carry only
'shift accountability' (see above) i.e. their role is essentially supervisory (or something similar, but not managerial). The head of the
ward or unit thus carries 'twenty-four-hour accountability'. The
latter is responsible for the assessment of junior night staff, helped
by contributions from senior night staff.

Second Possibility
Junior night staff are seconded for the period they are on night duty
to the managerial control of senior night staff. During this time they
are accountable only to night staff. The (day) head of the ward or
unit is accountable for the supplies, records system, and general
organization, of the ward, day and night but is not accountable for
the performance of junior staff on night duty. This is a 'two team'
system of working with collateral-relations between the day and
night-teams.

In discussion in one H.M.C. Group, in which the nursing services carried out in various hospitals were split into two main
divisions each under a P.N.O., different systems of night organization were proposed for each division. The first division was considered sufficiently compact geographically and of sufficient size
to warrant a separate night duty organization headed by an S.N.O.,
who would be supported by a number of nursing officers and charge
nurses. In the other division, because of the types of units involved
and its scattered geographical nature, it was decided to make the
senior night staff accountable to a superior in the day-time structure. For example, the night duty N.O. in one hospital would be
accountable to the S.N.O. who was also in charge of that hospital
by day.

The Relationship of Nurse Training to Service Nursing

We have carried out intensive fieldwork with the staff of nurse
training schools in four different Hospital Groups, and in each
the same main problems have been disclosed.
  The basic problem springs from the fact that trainees of the

school ('students' on three-year courses studying for S.R.N. qualifications, and 'pupils' on two-year courses studying for S.E.N.
qualifications) are not just trainees, ostensibly on 'training allow-
ances', but form in fact the great part of the labour force for the
provision of nursing services in wards and departments. Hence
the main problem, which is on the one hand to keep trainees on
various planned programmes of practical placements in wards and
departments, according to the logic and needs of their personal
development, and on the other to move nurses freely and rapidly
around to cover the depredations of staff sickness and leave as well
as the impact of unpredictable fluctuations in work-load. Thus
clinical instructors complained in one project that when they went
to wards to give practical tuition to their trainees there, they often
found to their consternation that, unknown to them, the trainees
had been moved to other wards, which were not likely to provide
the right kind of training experience.

In another project, the senior staff of the school of nursing pursued this issue so hard that at one stage in discussions they stated
their belief that the placements laid down for trainees should be
binding and not susceptible under any circumstances to change
by the officer in charge of allocations or the senior staff of the
service divisions. But might this leave the nursing service in an
intolerable position on occasion? Closer thought and discussion
showed that the more tenable statement[12] was as follows.

(1) Teaching staff had an absolute right to decide the *requirements*
for practical training placements, but not the actual allocations
themselves.
(2) Service staff had an absolute right to decide the *requirements* for
service, but again not the allocations themselves.
(3) Logically, decisions on actual *placements* must therefore be
collateral i.e. they must be mutually acceptable, or submitted for
resolution to the C.N.O. who was accountable for both nurse-
service and nurse-training.

In this particular project the general organizational picture was
as shown in Figure 7.5(a). Given the analysis above, it was felt
that the relationship of Allocations Officer, who was at that time a
subordinate of the P.N.O. (General Division), to the P.N.O. and

[12] This statement was finally agreed by all the senior staff concerned in the
project, as well as the Head of the Teaching Division and the C.N.O.

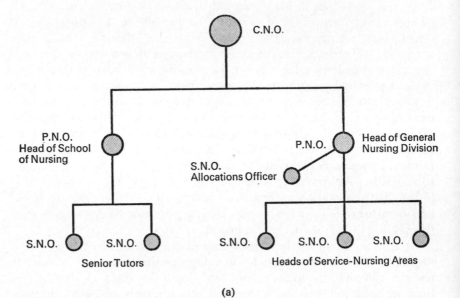

(a)

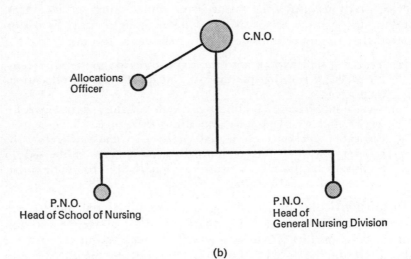

(b)

Figure 7.5

senior tutors in the School of Nursing could only be collateral. In the event of a disagreement about assignment, the two P.N.O.s might try to resolve the issue, again collaterally, and failing their agreement the issue would have to be referred to the C.N.O., who would have authority to settle the matter.

Later project-discussion suggested that it might be more requisite for the Allocations Officer to be directly subordinate to the C.N.O. herself.[13] In this way, he could more readily be seen to be taking an impartial stance between training and service requirements. At the same time, his relationship with both P.N.O.s (and their respective subordinates) could be a clear-cut staff relationship, so that only issues of major implication need be referred to the C.N.O. This would imply, of course, that the Allocations Officer had general policy guidance within which he could work. This could only come from the C.N.O., no doubt following discussion with the P.N.O.s in both the teaching and service areas.

A further implication of the recognition of the inescapable joint interest of teachers and service-nurses in the work and activities of trainees, is that the selection of trainees too, should logically be a joint matter.

Although the basic relationship of teaching staff and service staff is collateral, an additional feature must be added. The teaching staff in the same project saw themselves as having additional monitoring and service-giving relationships to service staff.

(1) It was seen as the duty of teaching staff to monitor the actual practical training received by trainees on the wards, and the nursing procedures being taught, to draw any deficiencies to the attention of the nurse in charge of the ward in the first instance, and failing satisfaction, to higher levels of the organization, for discussion. (See 'monitoring' relationship, Chapter 4.)

(2) It was seen as a duty of teaching staff to provide an advisory service, on request, in nursing procedures and techniques, to those service nurses who wished for technical guidance.

[13] This change has since been implemented.

Special Problems of Nursing at Small Hospitals

Work in one project with the heads of six small hospitals[14] has suggested that some special organizational problems may arise for nurses in these positions.

Even more than the ward charge nurse, the nurse in charge of a small hospital is general manager of a particular site. In addition to administering and co-ordinating treatment for in-patients the head may be accountable for organizing clinics or occasional theatre sessions, for maintaining a variety of medical and other records, for carrying out catering and cleaning, for ensuring the security and good condition of buildings and gardens, and even for some local 'public relations' work.

Because of this wide range of functions, the relationship between the nurse in charge and the central group administration is necessarily an important one. The Group Secretary may contact her directly on matters of public relations, or medical record systems, or establishment for ancillary staff, say; the Group Engineer and Building Supervisor may discuss repairs and rebuilding programmes with her; the Group Domestic Manager and Group Catering Manager will be closely concerned with cleaning and catering arrangements. How does all this fit with the apparent link with central nursing administration?

In this particular project it was in fact established that the link with nursing was predominant. It was confirmed that the nursing officers concerned were accountable to a more senior nurse (in this case the C.N.O.) and to her only. However it was also established that the Group Secretary, for example, would have a right to direct in matters of concern to him, but on the strict understanding that were his instructions to conflict with what the nursing officer concerned believed to be the policy or wishes of the C.N.O., she (the nursing officer) would refer the matter to the C.N.O., to resolve with the Group Secretary.

The nature of the relationships with other group heads has not yet been established in this project, but it was noted that two main possibilities exist.

(1) Group heads might play a central advisory and service-giving role (i.e. without any directive authority) for example, the Cater-

[14] The sizes in terms of beds ranged from 14 to 137. Three were 'general practitioner' hospitals.

ing Manager might supply certain foodstuffs on demand as a central service, or advise on purchase of new cooking equipment.

(2) Group heads might play a functional monitoring and co-ordinating role, with the right to give instructions to the nursing officer in relation to any group policies established within their particular fields, and the right to monitor the adherence of the nursing officer to group policies.

Finally, a special problem of relationship to medical staff was identified in the general practitioner hospitals. In these hospitals the beds were commonly available to all the general practitioners officially 'on the staff' of the hospital – some dozens in each case. As no one doctor was responsible for the use of beds, or indeed for his 'own' beds, the nursing officer in this situation was in the best position to review the general use being made of beds, and there-fore the suitability of any proposed admission of a patient. For example, one nursing officer pointed out that she would be much concerned to see that not too many beds at any one time were filled with chronic elderly patients – a situation which would change the whole nature and feel of the hospital, apart from its effect on future availability of beds. In consequence, she would certainly view with interest, and might at least discuss with the general practitioner concerned, the suitability of any proposed new admis-sion. The question, still unresolved, is: should she have the right to veto new admissions where she considered them totally unsuit-able in this way?

Conclusion

Our main finding as far as nurses are concerned, is that they are almost universally (if not universally) organized in hierarchies, under the management of one senior nurse, but subject to the treatment-prescribing authority of doctors. The main problem is to discuss exactly what internal structure is required in the nursing hierarchy in each situation, given that at least three kinds of roles – managerial, staff, and supervisory – are likely to be needed. Cer-tain units – separate hospitals, specialist divisions, and departments for example – suggest a clear location for certain managerial posts. The ward too, is probably such a 'natural' managerial unit, for the senior nurse in charge is not just the leader of a team of therapists, but a manager of all the operational services which bear on the patients in a particular site. Even more so is the nursing head of a small hospital a site-manager, and recognition of this fact leads to new thoughts about the relation between nurses and administrators, who (as we shall see in Chapter 9) have often a strong element of 'site-management' in their roles.

Note to Chapter 7

The Proper Role of the Nurse (page 121 above)

The proper role of nurses is a well-debated and long-debated question. It becomes even more difficult to answer when coupled with another question, one facing the Briggs Committee now sitting – namely, what varieties of training nurses need in order to carry out their role – since it undermines the obvious answer that nurses should carry out those activities, and only those, for which they are qualified by special training. (The Farrer Report (1968) for example took this line in defining non-nursing duties.)

Despite universal agreement that there should be activities identifiable as non-nursing activities, there is certainly little detailed consensus on which activities fall into which category. The Joint Working Party Report of the Royal College of Nursing and the National Council of Nurses of the United Kingdom and the Hospital Centre on Nursing Establishments (1966), suggests that: 'the ability to be jack of all trades and take on the role of others for the benefit of the patients is perhaps the new essence of nursing'. It emphasizes the general co-ordinating position of the nurse in relation to care of patients. 'Direct care and attention to the patients is given by medical staff, therapists, and technicians, as well as by professional and voluntary social and welfare workers. Because the ratio of patient to staff is greater in these fields, and because they do not expect to be in attendance throughout each twenty-four hours, these specialists depend upon nurses to assist, to continue with, to expand and complete their work.... Since trained nurses came into being they have taken the responsibility for the general welfare of patients in hospital wards and departments.' On the other hand, the Farrer Report talks of the enhanced 'therapeutic role of the nurse' which has evolved because of the rapid changes in diagnostic procedures and treatment techniques. The emphasis in that report is very much on the increased 'need for more technical nursing'. The Salmon Report (1966) steers a course mid-way between the two. 'Under the Nightingale pattern, catering, domestic cleaning, linen and laundry, and staff residences were usually placed in the Matron's sphere of authority. The current trend, rightly, is to relieve her of responsibility for them.

This is not to imply that nurses have no interest in their efficient functioning. On the contrary, on them depends the quality of the care that can be given by nurses to patients, as indeed on all the services that serve the purpose of the enterprise, such as building maintenance, engineering and others, which have not by tradition been placed under the Matron's control.'

8 Organization of Other Hospital Staff

One of the features of the development of hospital organization over the past century or so has been the evolution of a considerable variety of separate hotel-type and other general supporting departments which in earlier times formed an integral part of the work of the administrator or matron. In the middle of the nineteenth century, for example, the job of secretary at the Westminster Hospital included all the following duties 'to notify deaths, admit inpatients between house committee meetings, undertake fund raising, see that the hospital rules were maintained, dismiss unruly patients, visit wards daily, prevent smoking, visit kitchens, keep an eye on all provisions, supervise repairs and "attend to every department of the Hospital with vigilance, discretion and activity".'[1] The hospital matrons of the era were responsible not only for administering nursing services, but also for catering, domestic management, laundry, and linen — usually administered through assistant matrons.[2]

Present-day hospital organizations, however, see not only the existence of a wide variety of specialist posts in many of these fields at hospital level — supplies officers, engineers, building supervisors, domestic managers, catering managers and so on, but also a growing tendency for the formation of posts for group and even regional specialists[3] in the same fields.

[1] Abel Smith (1964, p. 32) (quoting Langdon-Davies, *Westminster Hospital — Two Centuries of Voluntary Service, 1719–1948*).

[2] Salmon Report (1966) Para. 2.10-2.14.

[3] Regional Engineers are well established. Regional Supplies Officers are coming into being following the Hunt Report (1966) on Hospital Supplies Organisation. The creation of Regional Building Officers is recommended by the Woodbine-Parish Report (1970) on Hospital Building Maintenance.

In this chapter we shall describe and analyse some of our find-ings from project-work about the organization of staff concerned with these services, at group and hospital level, services such as:

– engineering	– domestic	– medical records
– building	– catering	– medical secretariat
– supplies	– laundry and linen	
– C.S.S.D. (Central Sterile Supplies Department)	– porterage – telephonists – staff residences	

No one title seems apt for all these activities. The work is cer-tainly differentiated from medical, nursing, and paramedical, work in that it is not directly concerned with diagnosis or treatment for individual patients. The activities listed in the second column are often loosely described as 'hotel services' though again no strict definition of this term seems available in practice, and in any case this description does not happily fit all activities in the other two columns. Again, the activities in the third column seem different from the rest. Although medical records staff and medical secre-taries do not make decisions which directly affect diagnosis or treatment, they appear on the other hand to be more closely asso-ciated with the progress of individual patients than are staff carry-ing out activities in either of the first two columns listed above. So far, then, we have discovered no general categorization or descrip-tion here which will withstand the tests of logic or facilitate think-ing about how the activities concerned might be grouped organizationally.

Discussions in field projects with the staff themselves concerned in these fields have been limited for the most part to heads of department at hospital or group level.[4] Nevertheless all the

---

[4] Field projects have involved intensive individual discussions with about forty-six heads of departments from two teaching groups and six H.M.C. Groups, including five supplies officers, five building supervisors, three C.S.S.D. superintendents, five catering officers, six domestic superintendents, six group engineers, seven hospital engineers, one laundry manager, two linen-room heads, five medical records officers, and one head of medical secretariat; also (in domestic departments) with one deputy domestic super-

evidence from discussion has firmly indicated that the extant (not to
say requisite) nature of organization *below* the departmental head
level is basically hierarchical. That is to say, each departmental
head is in a full-managerial role, and fully accountable for the work
of all his staff. How many full-managerial levels lie below departmental head in various departments is another matter. Apart from
field project-work on the internal structure of domestic departments, our findings are limited so far to the results of conference
discussions. As far as these go, there is at least some evidence that
many of the more senior roles within hospital departments –
assistant engineers, building foremen, laundry charge hands,
kitchen superintendents etc. – are supervisory, rather than managerial, in nature.

So far, the main organizational problems revealed by field
project work in this area are:

(1) where each department as a whole fits into hospital organization,
and particularly, to whom the head of the department is accountable; and

(2) what is the nature of the relationship between group head of
specialist department and his counterpart at hospital level, and
the Hospital Secretary, where posts exist at both levels.

Relation of Head of Department to the Larger Organization

In very many situations explored in project-work we have found
great uncertainty amongst both departmental heads and associated
administrators as to where the department as a whole fitted into
the hospital organization. It can be expressed in one way as uncertainty about who the head of department is accountable to, or
in another way, as uncertainty about who, at the level of organization higher than that of departmental head, is accountable for the
general efficiency of the department and the morale of its staff. As
in the case of paramedical staff described in Chapter 6, many departments tend to 'float' organizationally; so that if things go badly
wrong (or what is more likely) do not evolve at the rate they should,

___

intendent, one senior supervisor, one area housekeeper and five ward housekeepers. However the issues unearthed have also been discussed with many
senior administrators and (in relation to domestic departments) with many
senior nurses from these eight Hospital Groups, as well, of course, as a wider
range of hospital staff in the conference-programme.

it is never quite clear who, above the level of departmental head, is to blame.

Broadly, this uncertainty is of two kinds. In some cases there is little doubt that the head is subordinate to the administration generally, the doubt being as to which individual administrator effectively acts as manager. We have found, for example, a Head of C.S.S.D. (Central Sterile Supplies Department), who on paper was accountable to an Assistant Group Secretary, but in practice felt that the Group Secretary himself was closer to being her true boss. We found an exactly similar situation for a Laundry Manager in relation to another Assistant Group Secretary. We found a Domestic Superintendent who was uncertain whether the Deputy Group Secretary or the Group Secretary was her immediate superior.

In these cases neither the departmental heads nor the administrators concerned were questioning the possibility of a departmental head being subordinate to an administrator. The real question could be seen to be that of selecting for each departmental head an administrator who would be of appropriate grade and ability to act convincingly as a real boss. More generally all the staff in the following fields with whom we have worked have readily seen themselves as ultimately subordinate to administrators at some level.[5]

- C.S.S.D.
- domestic

- catering
- laundry & linen
- porterage

- telephones
- staff residences (other than nursing heads)
- medical records
- medical secretariat

This leaves, from the list given earlier in this chapter, officers in engineering, building and supplies. It is in these fields that uncertainty of quite a different kind arises whether people in these fields are, or could properly be, accountable at all to administrators, however senior.

Now in relation to engineering and building, there is little

[5] It is worth noting that a D.H.S.S. Circular (Advance letter (AC) 4/70) has explicitly defined the direct accountability of occupants of two of the most senior posts in these fields – Group Catering Managers and Group Domestic Managers – to the Chief Administrative Officer of the H.M.C. or Board of Governors.

doubt that senior administrators are regularly and deeply involved in the general co-ordination of the work – for example, in moulding the formation of annual 'works programmes' and in monitoring the actual rate of progress in tackling such programmes. What many have doubted – Group Engineers particularly – is whether senior administrators do, or could appropriately play a full-*managerial* role in relation to them, with all its accompanying implications of rights (and attributes) to assess the work of the engineer in all its aspects, to prescribe work to be performed, in detail where necessary, and to help with work-problems encountered.[6] Often manifest evidence from a Whitley Council Circular (PTB 179) is cited, which describes a Group Engineer as 'the officer who is fully and directly responsible to ... an H.M.C.'. Building Supervisors on the other hand have been more inclined to see themselves as subordinate to the chief administrator, or even, in some cases, to his deputy; though in principle their situation would seem to be the same as that of engineers.

The situation for Supplies Officers is of a slightly different kind. In several places where we worked in the earlier stages of the project, the Supplies Officers saw themselves in reality as subordinate to senior administrators, even though on paper they were 'chief officers' of the authority (H.M.C. or Board of Governors) with the right of attendance at committees. The uncertainty here has arisen since the introduction of the ideas of the Hunt Report (1966) which proposed for the first time the setting-up of a larger supplies organization involving regional and area officers. The uncertainty now for Area Supplies Officers and Senior Supplies Assistants at H.M.C. Group level, is whether they are subordinate to the local Group Secretary or to the Regional Supplies Officer and Area Supplies Officer respectively, or to both in some degree.

---

[6] Again the general issue arises, discussed before in relation to both medical and paramedical staff, of the extent to which 'lay' administrators can appropriately manage, and be held fully accountable for, the work of professionals or 'semi-professionals'. As yet no decisive insight on this general question has emerged from the project, apart possibly from recognition of the peculiar organizational position of medical consultants (or any other independent therapists) which may arise by virtue of their special 'one-to-one' relationship with patients.

Organization at Group and Hospital Level

The other main organizational uncertainty for staff in these depart-ments arises where posts exist in the same specialty at both group and hospital level. This is frequently the case for example in engineering, domestic, catering, and medical records, departments. It is often the case too in certain of the paramedical specialties discussed in Chapter 6 – pharmacy, medical social work, and diet-etics, for example – and much of the following analysis applies equally well to them.

Before looking at these and other departments in detail it is helpful to consider certain organizational alternatives in a general way. Two main situations for any group head can be explored, those where the group head is directly accountable to the group chief administrator, and those where he is not.

Where the group head is subordinate to the group chief admini-strator, a pattern of relationships between group and hospital

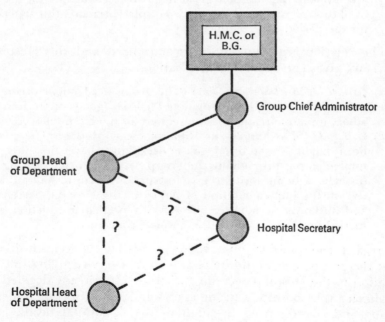

Figure 8.1   Possible Varieties of Two-Level Organization where the Group Head is Subordinate to the Group Chief Administrator

level arise as shown in Figure 8.1. The full lines from chief administrator to group head, and to Hospital Secretary, represent superior-subordinate relationships. The relationships to be explored are there shown by dotted lines.

The hospital head of department is obviously in a potential 'dual-influence' situation, and as described in Chapter 4 at least four varieties of relationship might be possible in such situations.

(1) *Outposting*. The hospital head might be subordinate to the group head, and in a position of having his work monitored for adherence to general discipline, local policies and regulations, and co-ordinated with that of other hospital officers by the Hospital Secretary. He might in addition be in a service-giving relationship to the Hosptal Secretary.

(2) *Attachment*. The hospital head might be co-managed by the group head and by the Hospital Secretary.

(3) *Functional Monitoring and Co-ordinating*. The hospital head might be subordinate to the Hospital Secretary, but subject to the functional monitoring and co-ordination of the group head.

(4) *Secondment*. The hospital head might be seconded by the group head (his original superior) to the Hospital Secretary (his superior for the period of secondment).

The relationship between the group head and the Hospital Secretary gives rise to further alternatives.

(1) *Group Head as Service Giver*. The group head might occupy a pure service-giving role, providing facilities (goods or services) or advice on request, and only on request, of the Hospital Secretary.

(2) *Group Head as Functional Monitor & Co-ordinator*. The group head might, in addition to service-giving, have the duty of implementing throughout the group agreed policies relating to his field, with authority to give instructions (akin to staff authority) on the implementation of policy to the Hospital Secretary, and authority to monitor the way his particular function was carried out in practice, in the hospital concerned.

As regards the combination of these alternatives, it seems unlikely that the group head would be restricted to a service-giving role in relation to the Hospital Secretary where it was already decided to establish a relationship as strong as attachment or functional monitoring and co-ordinating in relation to the hospital heads, and unnecessary to give him a functional monitoring and co-ordinating role where the Hospital Secretary was only receiving a service from an outposted departmental head who was already under his managerial control.

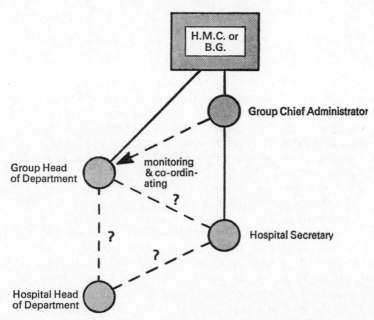

Figure 8.2   Possible Varieties of Two-Level Organization where the Group Head is Subordinate to the Governing Body

Where the group head is not accountable to the group chief administrator, but is accountable directly to the H.M.C. or Board of Governors the pattern of relationships to be considered is as shown in Figure 8.2. The relationship between chief administrator and group head, if not a superior-subordinate one, will probably be a monitoring and co-ordinating one, as will be suggested in the next chaper. The most likely rationale for the absence of a superior-subordinate relationship between the two springs from the nature of the specialty concerned. We must assume that the expertise necessary to pursue the specialty is such that it is unrealistic to expect a 'lay' person of whatever level of broad personal capacity, to play a full managerial role in relation to the head; that is, to be able to assess the work of the head of the specialty in all its aspects, and to be able to give effective prescriptions to the head on all matters, however technical.

If for the moment we assume that this reasoning is valid then we may comment on the possible relationships at lower level as follows:

(1) *Outposted service-giving.* This presents no difficulties as a possibility, as the managerial control rests with the technically-qualified group head.

(2) *Attachment.* This also is a possibility as it divides the operational control from the technical control, and gives the latter to the technically-qualified group head. However, the ultimate cross-over point in this 'co-management' situation is now no longer the chief administrator, but the governing body itself.

(3) *Functional Monitoring and Co-ordination.* This is unlikely, as it makes a 'technical' person (the hospital head) subordinate to a 'lay' person (the Hospital Secretary) in a way which is apparently considered impossible or at any rate inappropriate at the higher level.

(4) *Secondment.* This again is unlikely, for the same reasons.

As far as the relationship between group head and hospital head is concerned, again either *service-giving* or (more authoritative) *functional monitoring* and *co-ordinating* are still open possibilites, though in both cases the ultimate cross-over point, again, has shifted from chief administrator to governing body. As before, however, certain combinations of these alternatives with the alternative relationships to the hospital head are more likely to be workable than others.

'Group Advisers' at Hospital Level

All this assumes that the posts of group head and hospital head are quite separate. However, project-work has revealed a common situation where the group-head role is carried by an officer who is also the head of department in one particular hospital – often the largest hospital – in the group. For example, in a first move towards establishment of group control of medical records the most senior Medical Records Officer in the group, perhaps found at the largest hospital, may be given the title of Group Medical Records Officer. The problems which may arise in situations of this kind are exemplified in the following extract from a report on a project in a teaching group:

> Most of the Group Heads also occupied the role of Hospital Heads. Difficulty was experienced in distinguishing their two roles, and in establishing accountability as Hospital Heads of Departments. The principal trouble was in establishing what their relationship was to the Hospital Secretary and whether they spoke as Group Head of Department and as Hospital Head or not, and if not in what way the difference could be spelled out. The House Governor's double role as head of administration both in the Group and in the main hospital, made this problem yet more awkward to resolve. The difficulty in clarifying their own position at hospital level *vis-à-vis* the Hospital Secretary and the House Governor added to the Group Heads' difficulty in sorting out the nature of their relationship to department staff in the hospitals – it was not certain whether these were their own subordinates or those of the local Hospital Secretary; nor in either case what the relationship of department staff would be to the officer not in charge of them since both Hospital Secretary and Group Head had an interest in what hospital department staff did.

Subsequent work in this same teaching-group with the senior administrative staff and a number of departmental heads has produced the following general formulation for what has been called the role of *group adviser*.

> A group adviser is in subordinate relationship to a Hospital Secretary. The adviser may, however, be called upon from time to time by the House Governor or one of his subordinates, or by a committee, to give advice on the policy, budgets or work of that function for the whole Group;
> - the adviser must thus be authorized to visit other installations in the Group to keep informed about problems and developments;
> - he may have to attend meetings;
> - he may have to assist with the training of a new chief appointee in another hospital;
> - he may have to work full-time or nearly full-time for short periods in order to assist in such projects as the organization of another hospital.
>
> The adviser is not, however, managerially accountable for departments in any other hospital than his own.
> - he may offer suggestions to other departments but not issue instructions;

– he is not accountable for the staffing of other departments, but may be asked for advice on recruitment and selection problems.

With all these general problems and alternatives in mind we may now look more specifically, one by one, at what project-work has revealed so far in relation to the various specialties listed at the beginning of the chapter.

Engineering and Building

It is natural to look at engineering and building together, as the work of the two departments is so closely interlinked. In two situations at least, among those we have studied, the Building Supervisor is actually subordinate to the Group Engineer.[7] Where he is not, a strong mechanism for mutual operational co-ordination has to be established. Usually this is supplied by a senior administrator who agrees detailed work-programmes with both the engineer and builder, and subsequently follows the general progress of work.

As has been remarked, many (though not all) Group Engineers stress their direct accountability to the governing body, whereas Building Supervisors usually see themselves as subordinate to a Group Engineer or senior administrator.

As far as the two-tier organization of building and engineering work at group and hospital level is concerned, one early project explored the question in considerable depth in one group, with a

---

[7] The Woodbine-Parish Report (1970) claims (para. 4.2.3) 'In practice there exist four variants of the relationship between the Building Supervisor and the Group Engineer:
   (a) When the Group Engineer is responsible for all the duties carried out by the Building Supervisor;
   (b) Where the Group Engineer is not responsible for building mainten- ance work carried out by the Building Supervisor but is responsible for general co-ordination of building and engineering maintenance;
   (c) Where engineering and building maintenance work are undertaken in two separate departments, with the Group Engineer and Building Supervisor controlling their own staff; and
   (d) Where no Building Supervisor has been appointed.'
It goes on to recommend in the short term (para. 6.1.39) that 'the Group Secretary should be recognised as the non-technical co-ordinator of projects between the "clients" and the works organisation;' and in the long term (para. 6.3.3) 'the introduction of an integrated works organisation, covering both building and engineering maintenance under the supervision of the R.H.B.s.'

number of engineers, builders and administrators.[8] The result of
the first round of discussions was a conclusion that an *attachment*
relationship for engineering staff was the requisite one for this
particular Hospital Group, with the question left open as to
whether building work was better organized as a central service
under the Building Supervisor (who was a subordinate of the
Group Engineer) or carried out by staff at hospitals attached to the
Hospital Engineer or Hospital Secretary. It was remarked in a
summary report at this stage that:

> the essence of attachment is that Hospital Secretaries decide the
> priorities of work for Hospital Engineers, whilst the Group Engineer
> decides what training is needed for them and what standards to lay
> down within Group Policy.

However, later discussions suggested that a vital point had been
missed: that the operational programme for engineering and building work throughout a hospital group needs a high degree of
central planning and control. If this was right, attachment would
be quite wrong, and outposted service-giving the appropriate form.
Extracts from the final report on group discussions are worth quoting at length as an example of how an analysis of certain basic
features of a situation (in this case the nature of the work to be
carried out) may be used to indicate that one kind of organizational
relationship, rather than another, is requisite.

The Nature of Engineering and Building Work
Engineering and building work in the group consists of:
  (a) routine maintenance (eventually to be on planned preventive
      maintenance basis) called *maintenance*;
  (b) major and medium maintenance and installation projects,
      called *specials*;
  (c) *ad hoc* work which arises within hospitals and which can be
      carried out as and when maintenance and specials allow, called
      minors.

With respect to maintenance and specials, budgets and priorities
must be planned on a Group basis with a Group annual budget and
in the context of overall budgeting and priorities as advised by
Group Administration, Hospital Secretaries, and Heads of Departments. This central planning is necessary because the competing

[8] Including the senior administrators, Group Engineer, Building Supervisor, three Hospital Engineers and three Hospital Secretaries.

needs of the various hospitals cannot all be filled within available resources including the limited use of contractors.

A second characteristic of engineering and building work is the uncertainty of its progress. Starts may be delayed; delays inevitably occur while work is in progress: modifications are introduced; unforeseen problems arise. Overall programming must therefore also be centrally arranged so as to achieve the best distribution of resources at any given time. This distribution must be on a Group basis, since major modifications to the programme in any hospital, or in emergency, will affect the total Group maintenance and specials budget.

It is only the minors that can have priorities set at hospital level. The larger-scale Group works must, however, have priority over these. In the course of on-going projects and maintenance and specials it becomes possible to fit the minors into the on-going work programmes, but it is not possible to say precisely when a given minor can be carried out, since that depends upon the progress of the specials and on maintenance.

Establishment of Budgets and Programmes

In outline, it would follow that there must be a Group budget for maintenance and specials work. The Group budget shoud set out priorities and costs for the year's planned work; and would need to be modified as necessitated during the year by unforeseen difficulties, emergencies, failure of delivery, and other circumstances.

There would be a hospital budget for minors. How this budget, once agreed, would be spent (i.e. priorities among minors in each hospital) would be decided by the Hospital Secretary.

The Group Secretary would be accountable for finally approving the Group and hospital budgets and their on-going revisions for presentation to the Board. The Group Engineer would prepare the budgets and priorities, after discussion with other senior administrators concerned with development, hospital secretaries, the Building Supervisor, and hospital engineers. If Hospital Secretaries were not satisfied they would take the matter up with the Group Engineer and then the Group Secretary.

On specific projects, the Hospital Secretary would work out the brief in consultation with engineers. The brief once agreed by Group Secretary would be put into specification form say, by the Group Engineer.

The programming of on-going work would be arranged by Group Engineer. This would require close collaboration between Group Engineer and Hospital Secretaries accountable for the smooth running of the overall programme of activities in the hospital.

Outposting, Secondment and Attachment

If this analysis of engineering and building work is agreed, the organization required is the *outposting* of engineers and their staff to hospitals.

In addition to outposting, hospital secretaries get a *service* from engineers for carrying out minors. Where this work is likely to require a particular trade for, say, some months, the necessary tradesmen may be *seconded* to the Hospital Secretary, to be available to carry out the work the Hospital Secretary wants done under his own direction. If in fact the work is likely to keep a tradesman constantly employed full-time, then that tradesman can usefully be *attached* to the hospital secretary (as in the case of a carpenter in the medical school).

The particular group described above had a heavy burden of development work, and it may be that with other patterns of work other organizational forms are possible. Detailed projects in the same areas are at present under way in two further Hospital Groups. In one at least, a strong consensus is forming that they too, require outposted service-giving, rather than some form with weaker functional control.

Supplies

Discussions with three Group Supplies Officers in the time before the implementation of the Hunt Report (1966) proposals showed that each at that time saw himself as accountable to the group chief administrator. No conclusive findings about the organizational relationships of Area Supplies Officers and Supplies Assistants at individual hospitals, just introduced at the time of writing, have emerged, though discussions are in hand.

The supplies officer (whether graded as 'Area Supplies Officer', 'Deputy Area Supplies Officer' or 'Supplies Assistant') at any hospital is now in a 'dual-influence' situation in respect of the H.M.C. (in the person of its Group Secretary) on the one hand, and his immediate senior in the regional hierarchy on the other. As in so many cases of major organizational change in the hospital service, however, there is now considerable uncertainty as to how this dual-influence situation should operate. In the last resort, is the supplies officer now to regard as his boss the Group Secretary, or this new senior on the supplies side? At this stage it is only possible to point again to the variety of organizational possibilites exposed at the start of this chapter.

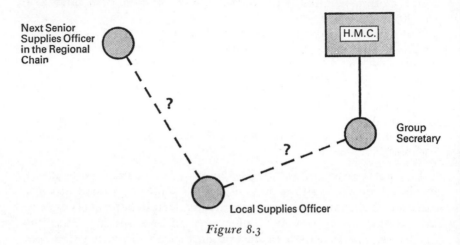

Figure 8.3

The chief possibilities again appear to be:

(1) outposted service-giving;
(2) attachment;
(3) functional monitoring and co-ordinating;
(4) secondment.

Given the underlying motive for reorganization, which was the believed need for a more centralized control of supplies work, it is difficult to see that secondment, at least, would be appropriate.

Central Sterile Supplies Departments

The job of central sterile supplies departments, as their name implies, is to provide packs of clinical instruments and materials (some disposable, others for re-use) sterilized and packed under controlled conditions, for use in wards, theatres and clinical departments. Our project-work has been limited to discussions with three C.S.S.D. superintendents plus a number of administrators who are concerned.

C.S.S.D. staff are fundamentally in a service relationship to nursing and medical staff. Within limits of agreed policies, they must supply what materials are demanded. Implicit in the service relationship, however, is the assumption that agreements to provide extended services, or new ranges of materials or instruments, require negotiation between the superintendent and the medical staff who are posing the new requirement. As C.S.S.D. staff normally see themselves as subordinate to administrators, any unresolved disagreement on services required or to be offered between a consultant and the superintendent would find ultimate cross-over point resolution only in the R.H.B. itself.

Associated with each C.S.S.D., by Ministerial direction, is a designated 'consultant with clinical responsibility for C.S.S.D.' – usually a pathologist. It appears from project-work that such consultants do not carry managerial roles in relation to C.S.S.D., as they sometimes do, for example, in relation to laboratory staff. They are seen as having definite authority, however, in relation to sterilizing methods, choice of equipment, tests, and standards of sterilization. Their role is probably best conceived as a combination of *advisory* and *monitoring* – with a duty to check on the standards actually reached, and ultimate right only to report unrectified shortcomings to the higher authority concerned.

Domestic Organization

As has been earlier observed, the trend over the years has been to remove from nurses a wide range of activities which could be conceived as 'non-nursing', for example laundry-work and catering. The management of cleaning in the larger hospitals has for many years been in the hands of domestic superintendents, formerly subordinate to the matrons, but now more usually to senior hospital administrators. However, even with the removal of laundry, catering, and cleaning, duties, a large number of activities remained to be carried out on the ward which did not evidently demand the specific skills of trained nurses – receiving phone calls, taking messages, carrying trays and crockery, preparing beverages, arranging flowers, maintaining linen stocks, etc.[9] Gradually a heterogeneous body of 'ward clerks', 'receptionists', 'ward aides' and 'ward assistants' grew up in order to relieve trained nurses of some of these

[9] A full list of these activities, based on systematic observations by the N.H.S. Central O & M Unit is given in Appendix IV of the Farrer Report (1968).

activities. The Farrer Report (1968) recommended that all these kinds of staff, together, in most cases, with cleaners, should be amalgamated into general-purpose ward housekeeping teams, and this recommendation has now been implemented in many hospitals.

We have been concerned in two major field projects in helping to define and clarify the various roles and relationships arising from the introduction of housekeeping teams. In both cases housekeeping teams have been envisaged as part of the domestic organization (this appears to be an assumption generally made, although not explicitly spelt out in the Farrer Report). At the same time, the Report suggests that individual teams should be 'seconded' to the sphere of authority of the ward sister, where 'secondment' is used in the sense precisely defined by the Salmon Report (1966) and thus invokes the notion of the 'sapiental authority' (sic) of the ward sister – the 'right to be heard by reason of knowledge or expertise'.

However, our own project-work has not indicated that such a definition is neither used, or if used, understood, so that real uncertainty still exists on many important issues such as the following:

- to what extent can the ward sister determine the work of the housekeeper?
- to what extent can she discipline her?
- to what extent is she responsible for her induction or training?

If a housekeeper stands on her rights, and refuses to carry out certain sorts of work demanded by the ward sister, what does the latter do next? Or if she thinks that the housekeeper is not suitable for her job, what can she do, if anything, to get her moved? Is this now entirely a matter for the domestic organization?

In the first of the two housekeeping projects in which we have been involved,[10] extensive discussions suggested that the requisite situation of housekeepers was what in this research has been called 'attachment' (see Chapter 4). This is in contrast to other possibilities, for example, 'outposted service-giving' or 'secondment' (here differently defined than in the Salmon Report – see again Chapter 4). The situation to be established was described in more detail in a project-report for one particular hospital in the terms quoted

[10] At Dulwich Hospital, in the King's Hospital Group – general report now published (*Nursing Times*, 1969).

below. (It should be borne in mind that in this particular hospital at the time concerned, the Domestic Superintendent was still accountable to the Matron and also that no significant organizational structure existed as yet between the level of Domestic Superintendent and Ward Housekeeper.)

> The ward housekeeper will have two superiors, who are together accountable for her work to their common superior, the Matron. The relationship is called *attachment*.

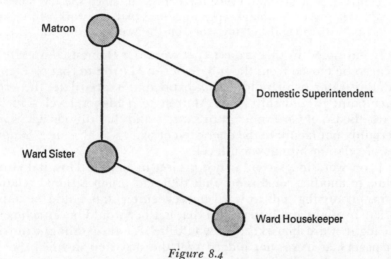

Matron

Domestic Superintendent

Ward Sister

Ward Housekeeper

Figure 8.4

Attachment assumes that the work done by the ward housekeeper has two components – operational (that is, what is to be done and when), and technical (how the task is to be done) – and that accountability for them can be separated. The operational superior (the ward sister) allocates tasks to the ward housekeeper, and the specialist superior (the Domestic Superintendent) instructs her on the method and techniques of executing domestic tasks, which constitutes a prescription on how the work is done. The prescriptions of how to carry out patient-care, of course, will be left to the sister.

Together the ward sister and the Domestic Superintendent have all the components of managerial authority in their respective areas over the subordinate, since together they are accountable for her work. They will together assess the performance of the housekeeper and would be able jointly to initiate her transfer. The Domestic Superintendent would not, for example, remove a housekeeper from a ward without consulting the sister. Both the sister and the Domestic Superintendent will jointly appoint the ward housekeeper for the pilot-scheme. (It has not yet been decided whether or not this will remain the practice.) This joint accountability assumes a *collateral relationship* between the ward sister and the Domestic Superintendent. In the case of disagreement over staffing, or assessment, they would refer the matter to the Matron, as the *cross-over point*, for resolution.

In the organizational arrangement of 'attachment' the ward sister retains overall accountability for her ward, since she has sufficient authority over the housekeeper to ensure that her work will be kept in line with general nursing work on the ward.[11]

It was noted in this project that were the Domestic Superintendent to be moved from the sphere of the Matron to that of a senior administrator (which did in fact happen at a later date) the 'cross-over point' would shift from Matron to a higher level – in fact to the Board of Governors in this case – and that this change would certainly not facilitate the operation of what was already a complex set of relationships at ward level.

Later work in a second major project in another Hospital Group came to another conclusion, that different organizational relationships of nursing staff to ward housekeeping staff would be appropriate by night and by day, and that neither would be 'attachment'. At night, ward housekeepers would be *seconded* to night nursing managers, as it was not judged that the situation justified the employment of senior housekeeping (domestic) staff in a supervisory or managerial capacity on night duty. For day duty, they would be in a situation of *outposted service-giving* to ward charge-nurses.[12]

The project was concerned not only with the work of housekeepers, but with the work of domestic staff generally throughout the group, referred to at the start of the project as 'ward aides' and 'senior housekeepers' in ward areas and 'domestics', 'domestic supervisors' and 'senior housekeepers' in non-ward areas. The important step was taken in the project of distinguishing the

[11] This description is not in fact totally different from the 'blow-by-blow' account of the proper operation of the principle of secondment in the case of ward cleaners as specified by the Salmon Report (1966) Appendix 8.

[12] It may perhaps be significant that in both domestic organization and engineering organization, situations which on first exploration seemed to call for *attachment* on second or deeper looks were judged to require *outposted service-giving*, with its implication of greater 'functional' control.

grades of staff employed from the *post title*, and both from the quite separate subject of *executive role*.[13] It was decided to use the appellation 'housekeeping' for all posts, and to establish a number of post-titles as follows:

> *In Ward Areas.*
> Senior Housekeepers.
> Ward Housekeepers.
> Housekeeping Aides.
>
> *In Other Areas.*
> Senior Housekeepers.
> Housekeeping Supervisors.

It was recognized that the grades to be attached to these posts were another matter.

Ward Housekeepers (in ward areas) and Housekeeping Supervisors (in other areas) would play a *supervisory* role in relation to their respective housekeeping aides, but the first full-managerial role would be at Senior Housekeeper level in both cases (Figure 8.5).

As far as relationships of housekeeping staff with charge-nurses or nursing officers were concerned, or with other local managers in sites other than wards, three different situations were discerned in the final report.[14] in keeping with the degree of involvement in housekeeping services likely to be required by these 'local managers'.

(1) In non-nursing areas, local managers (e.g. chief pharmacist, medical records officer) require little involvement. A straightforward *service-giving* relationship will be appropriate, in which the housekeeping organizations broadly provide the managers with cleaning services (within policy) which they require. It will be up to the local managers, as part of this relationship, to monitor the quality of cleaning service provided, but that alone.

---

[13] See discussion of these same distinctions in relation to nursing organization in Chapter 7.

[14] The final report, which incorporated material on retitling and general re-organization of domestic work (as indicated above), as well as more detailed material on the relationships of ward housekeepers to nursing staff, was agreed by the senior domestic, nursing and administrative staff in the Hospital Group concerned, and is now in process of being agreed with the Regional Steering Committee as a pilot re-organization project for implementation and test.

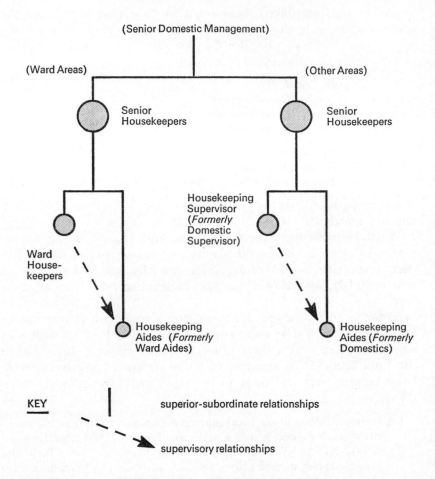

(Senior Domestic Management)

(Ward Areas)   (Other Areas)

Senior
Housekeepers

Senior
Housekeepers

Housekeeping
Supervisor
(*Formerly*
Domestic
Supervisor)

Ward
House-
keepers

Housekeeping
Aides (*Formerly*
Ward Aides)

Housekeeping
Aides (*Formerly*
Domestics)

KEY   superior-subordinate relationships

                            supervisory relationships

Figure 8.5   Organization of Housekeeping Staff in Wards and other Areas

(2) In nursing areas, where housekeeping staff are implementing work in close proximity to, or directly for the benefit of, patients, the local managers must be much more closely involved. At the same time, it is desired to leave the main weight of responsibility for management with the domestic organization. To achieve both these requirements an *outposted service-giving* relationship is the most appropriate.

Local nursing managers will:

(a) co-ordinate the particular tasks of ward housekeeping staff to meet the hour-by-hour needs of the ward, for example by rescheduling normal work-programmes, where necessary;

(b) assist in the induction of new staff into the ward situation;

(c) monitor to ensure that the activities of housekeeping staff conform to reasonable standards, discussing failures of standard with housekeeping staff in the first instance, but ultimately reporting them to the senior housekeeper;

(d) request specific services from ward housekeepers as required, of kinds defined by policy: e.g. help in serving food, taking of messages, etc.

Senior Housekeepers will:

(a) act as the managers of ward housekeeping staff, who are solely accountable to them;

(b) formulate their duties and lay down normal work programmes after consultations with appropriate nursing staff;

(c) select and allocate staff, and determine their transfer or dismissal, if needs be.

(3) The above will apply to day ward housekeepers. Night ward housekeepers will be *seconded* to appropriate senior nursing roles. The housekeeping organizations will provide staff recruitment and general staff administration, but housekeepers will be accountable, for the length of time they are seconded, to the senior nurse concerned.

Catering, Laundry, Linen, etc

It is generally accepted for catering, laundry, linen, portering, and telephone, services, and increasingly for the management of staff residences, that the staff concerned are, or can be made, fully accountable to administrators; and that administrators can and do act in full-managerial roles in relation to staff busy with these things. The main problem revealed by project work appears to be in finding the appropriate level at which to fit such departmental heads into the administrative organization in order that realistic and tenable relationships between supervisors and subordinates result. Sometimes quite junior departmental heads are apparently accountable directly to Group Secretaries or House Governors; on the other hand more senior departmental heads – catering managers for example – are sometimes apparently accountable to quite junior administrators.[15]

Medical Records and Medical Secretariat

Work with medical records staff has confirmed that they too see themselves as subordinate to administrators, and in a service-giving relationship to medical and nursing staff in such matters as arranging clinic visits and admission on request, and filing and removing medical records for use in clinics, theatres, and wards, on request.

The types and forms of medical records to be maintained are requisitely a matter for negotiation with medical staff. Medical Records Committees are often formed to discuss these matters, manned by consultants selected by medical committees, and attended by medical records officers. Project-work has revealed at least one situation where the consultants effectively establish, through a 'medical records sub-committee', their own policy on records, unilaterally; but it would appear requisite that proposals for change in records should not become accepted as established policy unless approved by the governing body concerned, or one of its officers on its behalf, the medical records officer in the first instance.

However, medical records departments not only maintain records, but commonly also provide reception and general information services to the public. If these latter activities are regarded as part of the operational functions of the hospital (and we shall argue in Chapter 10 that they are) then it would appear that in respect of these activities medical records departments act collaterally or in collaboration with doctors, nurses and others who also carry out operational functions.

Medical secretarial services are closely related to all these activities, and indeed in many hospitals medical records and medical secretariat are combined under one head. Project discussions have

[15] We are at present attempting on one project to get some measure of the varying levels of work arising for heads of these and other departments in order to form a systematic basis for deciding which naturally fit 'high' and which 'low' in any organization, using the time-span measure developed by Jaques (1967), but results are not yet available for general publication. It is probable that the role of some of the more junior administrators – supposedly in the full-managerial chain – is not managerial at all, but co-ordinatory or supervisory only.

suggested two possibilities for the organizational location of the individual secretaries themselves:

(1) they might be service-giving to doctors, in a central pool managed by one head secretary – or
(2) they might be individually seconded, for various periods of time, to work for individual doctors, to whom they are then temporarily accountable.

Conclusion

To reiterate, the main organizational problems associated with these various supporting services are not, so far as can be seen, about the internal structure of individual departments, but about the relationship of the head of the department to the local chief administrator and (where he exists) to the corresponding group officer in the same function.

In many functions the possibility of subordination to administrators (at some level) is seen as realistic, but in others, notably engineering, there is considerable doubt.

Whatever the outcome of this question, however, the growth of group and even regional posts in these fields is placing more junior officers in a situation of dual-influence – local, and functional – and although a rich variety of choices of structuring these difficult dual-influence situations is possible, little of real substance in the way of definition appears to have been achieved so far in the service.

9 The Role of Administrators and Finance Staff

In the early stages of project-work, the role of the administrator seemed particularly impervious to exact analysis and definition. The analogy of the commercial chief executive was not helpful, and indeed positively misleading in some ways, and yet at the same time the senior administrator seemed to have a breadth of concern for his hospital or group as a whole that paralleled the concern of the commercial chief executive for every part of his own enterprise. Impressionistically, one felt that the presence of administrators was like a cement that bound the whole hospital organization together, so that wherever a crack appeared in the structure, however high or low, under good administration at least the cement smoothly flowed and filled it.

Administrators were the co-ordinators, the middle-men, the fixers. They were in some ways, to the hospital or group as a whole, what the charge nurse was to the individual ward. But whilst the breadth of their activities was evident, the exact nature of their authority was uncertain in the extreme.

The role of the chief administrator (Group Secretary or House Governor) in providing conventional secretarial services for his committee (H.M.C. or Board of Governors) was an easy and obvious starting point for definition, but we soon gathered from those chief administrators with whom we worked that this secretarial role was in some ways the lesser part of their job. What were the additional functions? What relationship did they engender between the chief administrator and other chief officers – that of a superior or that of a collateral colleague?

The Role of the Chief Administrator

Gradually, a coherent and reasonably consistent formulation of the role of the chief administrator has emerged from project-work.[1] Here is a typical statement from work with one Group Secretary, agreed with him as an accurate reflection of his role.

In general terms, the Group Secretary sees himself as carrying two closely associated roles:
– secretary to the H.M.C., and
– chief executive officer of the Group.
As *secretary to the H.M.C.* his functions include such things as:
– ensuring that arrangements are made for H.M.C. meetings, providing agendas and papers;
– keeping the H.M.C. informed of all statutory requirements and all policy requirements of the D.H.S.S. and R.H.B.;
– ensuring that minutes of all meetings are provided, and that appropriate individuals or bodies are informed of H.M.C. decisions, new or proposals.
As *chief executive officer of the Group* he has concern with every activity undertaken within the Group, by whatever section of staff, and concern with all relationships with the public, the R.H.B. and other bodies. As described below, he feels direct accountability for the provision of certain services (e.g. domestic services, catering, laundry, medical records and secretariat, transport and reception, and messenger service) through the medium of staff that are, extantly if not manifestly, his own *subordinates*. For the remainder, his role takes the form of a co-ordinating and monitoring function in relation to the activities of medical, nursing, and other, staff of the hospital. More specifically, this function involves him in the following types of activity:
– Ensuring that all H.M.C. decisions and policies are translated into action, by setting objectives and drawing up programmes of implementation, where necessary, and initiating action with all those concerned:
e.g. – arranging the introduction of new hospital facilities, involving new buildings, equipment, staff, and procedures;
– ensuring completion of special expenditure programmes.
– Ensuring that all essential services are maintained by developing appropriate control systems, by monitoring, and by taking what-

[1] Based on individual discussion with seven Group Secretaries and three House Governors; also on conference discussion with another dozen or so Group Secretaries.

ever corrective action is possible whenever a lapse appears imminent.
- Monitoring the activities of all hospital staff to ensure their adherence to general policy (or normal practice in the area where there is not explicit policy); discussing any deviations or adverse tendencies with the staff concerned and, if necessary, reporting such deviations to the H.M.C., or directly to the R.H.B.;
  e.g. – monitoring complaints;
        – monitoring waiting lists, bed usage;
        – monitoring all expenditure against budget.
- Initiating at his own discretion proposals for developments or improvements in standard, or the meeting of new needs in respect of any aspects of the work of the hospital;
  e.g. – discussing with the medical staff and the head of nursing possibilities of introduction of progressive patient care;
        – suggesting possibility of regular inter-disciplinary case-conferences for mentally sub-normal patients.
- Participating in the selection of all senior H.M.C. staff.
- Helping to induct new senior H.M.C. staff, or senior medical staff, into their working situation.
- Helping the H.M.C. to form assessments of the personal capacity of all senior H.M.C. staff. (In practice, informal reports would be made, where required, to the H.M.C. Chairman, rather than to the full H.M.C.).

This Group Secretary then (and he is typical in this respect of many others involved in the project) saw himself as in a superior-subordinate or managerial relationship to certain staff, and in monitoring and co-ordinating relationship to the remainder. Now, in many ways, the same sorts of functions are carried out in each of these relationships. The detailed functions listed in the extract above are broadly similar to the generalized list of managerial functions given in Chapter 4. The most significant differences are that the Group Secretary, in carrying out monitoring and co-ordinating functions in relation to those whom he co-ordinates:

(a) need not have a veto, or indeed any part in appointment;
(b) will not usually have any authority to instruct in what would be regarded as technical matters;
(c) would have no authority to make formal assessments, to initiate transfer or dismissal, or in any way to sanction;
(d) must accept the right of direct access of those co-ordinated to the person or body to whom they are in the end accountable – in this case the H.M.C.

The most difficult thing is to decide just what degree of authority the chief administrator does carry in his monitoring and co-ordinating role. Ultimate sanctions rest wholly with the employing body (though these are of course, limited in all cases and particularly in the case of consultant employees, as described in Chapter 5). Nevertheless his words have on occasion the force of prescription, rather than just advice. The recipient cannot ignore them at will, but must persuade the chief administrator to another view, or else either act on the prescription, or cause the matter in dispute to be referred to the governing body for resolution. This implies of course that the governing body itself carries authority in the matter. If it does not, then the chief administrator cannot give instructions, as it were, on behalf of that body. Thus a chief administrator could not in his co-ordinating role give instructions to a consultant on clinical matters with even the limited degree of authority described above, since the governing body who employed the consultant (the R.H.B. or Board of Governors) could not do so either.

In relation to certain staff, however, the chief administrator carries full-managerial authority; certainly in relation to his own deputy, assistants and clerical staff, and commonly to staff in many supporting services, such as medical records, catering, and domestic departments, as described in the last chapter.

So far, project-work has not been able to establish any definite or well-established line of division between those departments in relation to which the chief administrator carries full-managerial authority and those in relation to which he carries only monitoring and co-ordinating authority. Borderline cases apparently include engineers, builders and various heads of paramedical departments. It has even been suggested that managerial relationships appertain in reality between chief administrators and chief nurses and treasurers in certain hospital groups.[2] Doctors, however, in our project-

---

[2] In the absence of clear and public concepts of managerial and co-ordinating roles, given the central position of the chief administrator, all turns on his individual influence, personality and prestige, in relation to other particular individual officers. There is little doubt that certain relationships of the chief administrator in some Hospital Groups have all the psychological feel of full-managerial ones, whilst these same relationships in other Groups are no stronger than collateral, in effect, given the particular personalities involved. The role of chief administrator in its present undefined state, is more capable than most, of extension or contraction at will.

work, have always been seen as beyond the line of possible managerial relationships.

In the same project-report mentioned above the relation of the Group Secretary to medical staff, as he perceived it,[3] was described as follows:

> The Group Secretary perceives himself as expected to carry out in relation to medical staff most of the co-ordinating and monitoring functions listed above.
>
> He might on appropriate occasion, be expected to have discussions on any of the following topics, for example, with any member of medical staff:
> (1) the doctor's own attendance record;
> (2) any possible question of unprofessional or negligent behaviour, or personal incapacity;
> (3) length of waiting lists;
> (4) use of beds;
> (5) number of patients dealt with per session;
> (6) drug usage;
> (7) possible changes in session times, or session arrangements;
> (8) allocation of space, equipment, beds or services, to the doctor concerned.
>
> The Group Secretary would clearly not be acting in a superior-subordinate relationship in such matters. To repeat, he would be acting as a general co-ordinator and monitor of medical services on behalf of the H.M.C., who themselves have this duty. His authority would be limited to:
> – authority to make interim rulings on level of services to be made available to medical staff or on session times for them, subject to the right of referral to H.M.C.;
> – authority to discuss any of the topics (1) to (6) above, with a view to securing developments or improvements, but no authority to insist on such changes, even pending referral to the H.M.C.
>
> In the event that the Group Secretary believed that a doctor was acting outside the bounds of acceptable behaviour in respect of any of these activities, and had been unable to persuade him to return within bounds, he would have a choice of referring the matter for further action to:

---

[3] Whether his medical colleagues in the same hospital group would accept the following formulation in all its detail, is not at this stage known. Certainly it would be interesting to explore with them how much, if any, of this monitoring and co-ordinating work ought in the first instance to be carried out by medical committees or their chairmen.

- the H.M.C. (or its Chairman);
- the local Medical Staff Committee (or its Chairman);
- the Group Medical Advisory Committee;
- the standing medical committee concerned with incapacity of individual doctors;
- the S.A.M.O. at the R.H.B.

The Group Secretary is not, however, concerned with the selection of senior medical staff, or with helping to form any assessment of the personal capacity of members of medical staff, other than in the extreme case mentioned above.

Hospital Secretaries

Work with a large number of hospital secretaries[4] reveals almost exactly the same picture in miniature as for group administrators. The Hospital Secretary does not normally act as secretary for a hospital committee (following the decline of 'house committees') as does the chief administrator of the Group, but he too is concerned with the complete spectrum of activities in his unit. He too carries on accepted full-managerial role in relation to certain categories of staff – clerical staff, porters, cleaners and the like – and some degree of monitoring and co-ordinating role in respect of all other staff in the hospital. Again, there are many borderline cases where the extant presence or absence of a full-managerial relationship is often in doubt – in engineering and certain of the paramedical specialties for example.

The great problem for Hospital Secretaries, as so many have expressed it to us, a problem which does not as yet bear to the same extent on group chief administrators, is that of maintaining a credible role in the face of increasing 'functional management'. With the appointment of Group Domestic Managers, Group Catering Managers, Group Medical Records Officers, and so on, the Hospital Secretary is increasingly stretched between his continuing feeling of responsibility for the work of his hospital in all its totality, on the one hand, and his clear recognition of diminishing or diluted authority on the other.[5] Many aspects of this situation

[4] About 23 Hospital Secretaries have been involved in individual discussions in field-projects in addition to a further large number in conferences.

[5] Cooper (1971) has analysed this erosion of the Hospital Secretary's role in some detail and suggested the need for the explicit recognition of the role of Hospital Secretary as 'integrator' (in the language of Lawrence and Lorsch

have of course been touched on in the previous chapter, where the Hospital Secretary was seen as a regular party in 'dual-influence' situations.

The extent of the monitoring and co-ordinating authority of the Hospital Secretary in relation to medical staff is more uncertain than that of the Group administrator in relation to the same doctors. No doubt status and personal weight come into this, and there must clearly be some point at which the monitoring and co-ordinating role loses credibility in face of the inverse status of the co-ordinator and those whom he seeks to co-ordinate. On the other hand, as always, what is implicit and unrecognized is never quite as potent as what is explicit and accepted. The following comments were recorded after discussion of the nature of their roles with three Hospital Secretaries from one H.M.C. group.

It is necessary to emphasize about co-ordinating and monitoring authority (in this situation) that it exists spontaneously, but is not explicit, i.e. has not so far been described, defined and set up as a matter of policy by the H.M.C. It cannot therefore be referred to as a tool to help those who feel they carry it to use it effectively.

Thus, for example, the nature of the Hospital Secretary's authority in relation to junior medical staff is not currently easy for all concerned to specify; the Hospital Secretary who brings pressure to bear on a junior doctor to attend a clinic (so that the Hospital Secretary can ensure that an adequate outpatient service is provided in terms of cover, hours and so forth) must therefore do so on the basis of whatever personal resources and various devices are open to him, rather than on the basis of authority assigned to him specifically to do that job.

If this analysis is correct, its status is not simply that of a recommendation; it describes what exists in the working situation and what attempts are being made by individuals operating in that situation to carry out effective work.

What individuals can do by their own efforts is however different from what they can do once their authority is explicitly stated to all concerned. In other words, once the co-ordinating and monitoring role, its accountability and therefore its authority were all clearly stated, Hospital Secretaries would be enabled to do more than can be done at present to review effective overall running, seek the best

---

(1967)) as well as representative within the hospital of the 'institutionalized system', i.e. the link with the community, the values it sets, and the resources it provides.

overall solutions to day-to-day matters, propose necessary changes in policy or point out lack of policy.

Whatever their precise view of their role within their own hospital, however, all the Hospital Secretaries with whom we have worked see themselves as accountable to the Group Secretary, and to him only, for everything they do.

Deputy and Assistant Secretaries

Although Deputy Group Secretaries and other assistants at group level are clearly subordinate to Group Secretaries, and Deputy Hospital Secretaries to Hospital Secretaries, it is difficult to generalize about the specific functions[6] of any of these deputies and assistants. In practice they tend to be used in a fairly *ad hoc* way to assist their respective principals in all branches of work that the latter have to carry out. They help, for example, by taking notes of meetings, by carrying out special information-collection activities or surveys, by maintaining personnel records, by working out detailed schemes for new administrative procedures or new organization, and by progressing the implementation of new developments of all kinds. Over and above this they may help their principal – shadowing him as it were – in all his activities of monitoring and co-ordinating, or in some cases, in managing the work of other staff of the hospital. Individual assistants and deputies in Groups or hospitals do usually indeed get assigned specific functions as a regular part of their work, but no one pattern of assignment seems to be universal or even predominant. The possible exception is a tendency for Deputy Group Secretaries to be specially concerned with the programming and progressing of building maintenance and development of all kinds.

However, looking generally at the question, the various ways in which help may be given to the chief administrator appear to be analysable in terms of the following categories:

(1) *Secretarial Work* – helping to arrange meetings, produce agenda, minutes, communicate committee decisions;

[6] The material of this section is based on project-discussion with six Deputy Group Secretaries, three Deputy House Governors, three Deputy Hospital Secretaries, two personnel officers, and about twenty assistant secretaries and administrative assistants, as well as with the Hospital Secretaries or Group chief administrators for whom they work.

(2) *Public Relations Work* – dealing with press, visitors, enquiries, and complaints;

(3) *Deputizing* – standing-in in the absence of the principal to make urgent decisions in any matter to which he would normally attend;

(4) *Personnel Work* – basically, maintaining personnel records, arranging recruitment, dealing with individual questions of pay and conditions of service; possibility of extension to broader topics; training, union and staff negotiations, organization-planning and development;

(5) *Departmental Co-ordination or Management* – co-ordinating, or alternatively managing (with full-managerial authority), the current operational activities of various specific hospital departments, or co-ordinating the development of these activities.[7]

Engaging in these different activities would imply the adoption of various types of organizational relationships to other staff of the hospital. Personnel work suggests a staff-officer role (see Chapter 4) with definite authority to implement agreed plans and policies. Deputizing would imply a partial taking-over of the role of the principal (see also Chapter 4) with certain of the prescriptive authority of that principal. (In the *presence* of the principal, the 'deputy' might carry out any of the other activities listed, or might act – and commonly does – as a sort of 'general staff officer' whether or not this is finally requisite as an organizational solution.) Departmental co-ordination would imply a monitoring and co-ordinating role and departmental management, a full managerial role.

Functional and Geographical Organization of Administrative Staff

At the present phase of project-work we are engaged in separate discussions with a number of chief administrators to establish for each what is the optimum form of administrative organization for his own local circumstances. In these discussions the following important principle has become clear. *In establishing a subordinate organization to help him administer and co-ordinate the work of a hospital group, the chief administrator will probably need staff organized both on a functional and on a geographical basis.* Neither geographically-organized, nor functionally-organized assistants

[7] See the further and broader discussion of the organizational division of operational and other (non-operational) activities in Chapter 13.

alone are likely to do the trick, apart from the special case of the one-hospital group.

The staff primarily concerned with the total administration of particular sites are, of course, the hospital secretaries (noting the apparent anomaly of the 'site-management' of small cottage hospitals by nursing administrators mentioned in Chapter 7). With the growth of functional management, as we have noted, the role of the local administrator has inevitably altered, and perhaps in some respects weakened, but we have received no evidence at all from this project that local administrative roles in geographically separate hospitals might be done away with altogether. The real need is to evolve an appropriate pattern of organizational relationships between local departmental head, group head, and local administrator, as discussed in Chapter 8, as various functional links between group and hospital are added.

At the same time, the enlargement in the numbers and varieties of specialist officers at group level has perhaps developed the need for a strengthened central administrative staff also organized along functional lines to underpin and co-ordinate the specialist services. In many of the larger hospitals we have encountered in project-work there is indeed no Hospital Secretary by that title. The chief administrator is usually in fact the local site co-ordinator, and his assistants and deputies tend each to be concerned with particular functions or groups of functions in that particular hospital, as well as in others.

Combining the requirements for both local and functional elements of the kind described above, a general model for administrative organization within the hospital group is illustrated in Figure 9.1.

Not all the posts shown would be necessarily separately established, indeed in smaller groups it is certain that many would be combined. Separately established personnel officers are still rare. In any case the deputy post cries out for combination with some other, as strictly speaking the role only has definite content in the absence of the chief administrator. One possible embodiment for a smaller group might be as shown in Figure 9.2 where the deputy would act as co-ordinator or manager of the general service and hotel-service departments, and the chief administrator himself would act as co-ordinator of medical, paramedical and nursing services. In carrying out these managerial or co-ordinating roles,

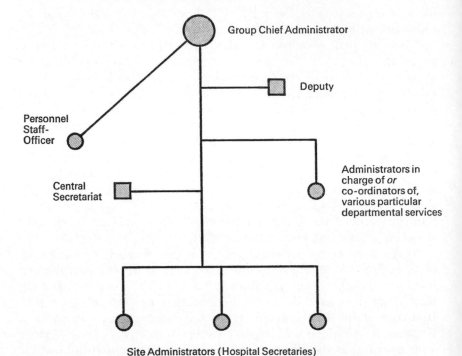

Group Chief Administrator

Deputy

Personnel
Staff-
Officer

Central
Secretariat

Administrators in
charge of *or*
co-ordinators of,
various particular
departmental services

Site Administrators (Hospital Secretaries)

Figure 9.1   A General Model for Group Administration

the chief administrator very likely would require assistance in the
shape of assistant secretaries or clerical officers – as might also the
deputy for his work. Such assistants might well share in the monitoring and co-ordinating work of their principals, for example, by
collecting and disseminating information, though without necessarily having the full authority of a monitor and co-ordinator. For
example, they might specifically not have authority to call co-
ordinating meetings or authority to discuss shortcomings in
standard. On the other hand they might in certain cases play a
full-managerial role in relation to certain smaller departments, for
example, linen rooms or porters.

The Role of the Treasurer
According to legislation[8] a hospital authority shall appoint a
Chief Financial Officer whose duties shall include the giving of

[8] Statutory Instrument 1969 No. 1582.

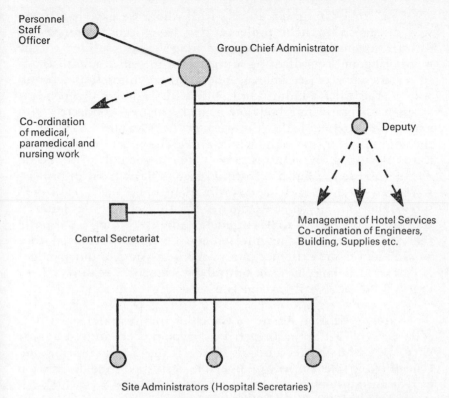

Personnel Staff Officer

Group Chief Administrator

Co-ordination of medical, paramedical and nursing work

Deputy

Central Secretariat

Management of Hotel Services Co-ordination of Engineers, Building, Supplies etc.

Site Administrators (Hospital Secretaries)

Figure 9.2   One Possible Example of Specific Group Administration

information and advice to the authority or any of its committees. Legislation allows the appointment of a joint group secretary and chief financial officer but in England at any rate[9] it is more common to appoint separate (Group) Treasurers as chief financial officers. Thus legislation sets the stage for a situation in which the governing body has direct access to financial advice and information, independently of the officers whose work incurs the bulk of the expenditure concerned.[10]

[9] Joint appointments are still the rule in Scotland according to Farquharson-Lang (1966 – para. 195) and according to them it is desirable that the function should continue to be brought together under one head (paras. 221-224).

[10] This situation is after all, usual in social organization. Voluntary associations regularly elect treasurers in addition to 'secretaries' who in that context act as chief executive officers. Commercial organizations appoint

Of the three Group Treasurers with whom we have had intensive discussion in field projects, two have seen themselves as directly accountable to their governing bodies, subject to the monitoring and co-ordinating authority of the chief administrator in certain respects (see below). The third saw himself as accountable to the chief administrator, but with right of independent access to the governing body on financial matters connected with audit. The problem is that the work of the Treasurer, like that of the administrator, spans the whole organization, and is concerned, again like that of the administrator, with control and co-ordination in a general sense. But how, administrators have asked in project-work, can there be genuine co-ordination unless the Treasurer is subordinate to one chief executive, whether or not the latter is trained in finance as well as general administration? Accepting that one means of genuine internal audit is thereby removed, they would point to the existence in any case of a system of independent audit conducted by officers of central government. Treasurers, however, do not necessarily accept this view.

If the only organizational possibilities appear to be for the Treasurer to be subordinate to the chief administrator or to be a collateral colleague, the breach in viewpoint does indeed appear wide. But with the recognition of the reality of monitoring and co-ordinating roles the way is opened to a third possible description of relationships between administrators and Treasurers which has seemed requisite (at least in terms of present hospital organization, regardless of whether it might be ideal in some more radical reconstruction) to a number of representatives of both groups of staff with whom we have worked.

This particular description (see Figure 9.3) allows that the chief administrator has a prime responsibility for the general monitoring and co-ordination of the work of the group, and that it would therefore be a proper part of his role to consider such things as the staffing and accommodation of the Treasurer's department, adherence to general hospital policies and customs, and production of financial data and advice in accordance with the needs of more general programmes. At the same time, the Treasurer would not in any sense be accountable to the chief

'secretaries' who are often responsible amongst other things for the production of accounts, in addition to managing directors who are in this second context the chief executive officers (Gower 1957, Chapter 1).

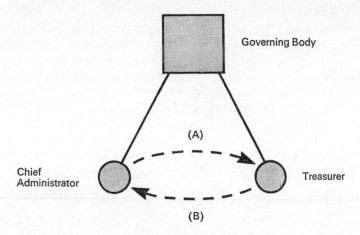

(A) – general monitoring and co-ordinating

(B) – financial monitoring

Figure 9.3

administrator – if we restrict the use of accountability to a relationship backed by assessment and sanction (see Chapter 4). Although the chief administrator would have *co-ordinating authority* in relation to the Treasurer, the Treasurer would be *accountable* only to the governing body who appointed him. This of course necessarily implies the right of direct access to the governing body by the Treasurer. In a project in one hospital group it was accepted by all the chief officers concerned[11] (including the Treasurer) that one of the duties of the Group Secretary would include:

> normally, collating and editing all reports, proposals and estimates for submission to the H.M.C., subject to the right of other Chief Officers to make direct submissions of their reports where there are important differences of opinion on content or presentation which have not been able to be resolved.[12]

[11] The project included the Group Secretary, the Treasurer, the Chief Nursing Officer and the Medical Administrator. After many months of discussion, individually and in small groups, a precise formulation was finally agreed from which the following extracts are taken.

[12] This formulation coincides perhaps with one interpretation of the proposal of the Bradbeer Report (1954) that 'all principal officers at group

Also in this same project, the Treasurer was seen to have a monitoring role on behalf of the H.M.C. in relation to expenditure, which was ultimately independent of the Group Secretary, although it was recognized that the latter too was concerned with monitoring rates of expenditure. The precise division of function between the two, and other chief officers (such as the Chief Nursing Officer) in regard to the control of expenditure was agreed to be as follows:

Extantly, the Group Secretary, other chief officers and the Treasurer are all concerned in various ways with control of expenditure. The following division of function is requisite:

It is the function of the *Treasurer* to record and publish actual expense data;

- note adverse trends in expenditure, discuss possible corrective action directly with the chief officer concerned, and advise on the financial implication of such action;
- where he was not satisfied that any action proposed was likely to correct the financial position, refer the matter to the Group Secretary for further action;
- where he judged that the action proposed would not have the effect of correcting the financial position, refer the matter to the H.M.C.

It is the function of each *Chief Officer* to take action within the limits of his authority where he judges it necessary in response to information on expense presented by the Treasurer.

It is the function of the *Group Secretary* within his overall monitoring and co-ordinating role, as defined above, to take whatever action in relation to other chief officers to control expenditure he judges necessary, normally in response to an approach by the Treasurer as described above.

Generally the right of the Treasurer to determine expenditure, either at the stage of preparation of budgets and activities, or at the later stage of control of rates of actual expenditure has been

---

level should in our view be responsible to the governing body *through* the chief administration officer ...' (para. 181). This Report, (in contrast to Farquharson-Lang) also notes the special arguments in favour of having a separate chief financial officer accountable directly to the governing body: 'we feel ourselves obliged to adopt the principle that it is undesirable to combine in the hands of one officer responsibility for spending public funds and responsibility for accounting for them' (para. 183).

seen as a difficult question. Clearly the Treasurer has *influence* in these matters: does he have *rights* to make final decisions? Logically he cannot, unless authority to use resources is to be separated from accountability for results. In the same project a further statement on the role of the Treasurer which covered this matter was produced and agreed:

> It is agreed that the Treasurer should in a general sense be regarded as part of the top management team of the Group. He should participate in policy formulation and he needs to be aware of all major policy decisions or proposals if he is to do his work effectively. This still leaves, however, the need to discriminate the role of the Treasurer in expense control from that of other chief officers, and particularly from that of the Group Secretary. The general implication of the precise divisions of function listed above, is that whilst the Treasurer's role certainly involves much more than the simple recording and publication of expense data it is not part of his role to decide by himself where or whether expenditure should be curtailed in any area. Requisitely it is the job of those with accountability for provision of service (output) to make decisions on where expenditure (inputs) should or should not be made, within the limits of their own authority.

Conclusion

The general conclusion from project-work is that, extantly, the administrator is neither the solely-accountable chief executive of the hospital, on the analogy of the industrial 'managing director', nor is he simply the managerial head of one particular group of service-departments, the old-time 'steward', working collaterally with other officers. His role is a complex one. It combines acting as committee-secretary, and as head of certain hotel and general services, with seeing as far as possible that all hospital activities are co-ordinated and developed as a whole. This latter duty brings him into a monitoring and co-ordinating relationship with his fellow chief officers, a relationship which broadly accords with his commonplace designation as 'first among equals', but which is capable of a precise definition which enables it to be distinguished from a collateral role on the one hand, or a full-managerial role on the other.

10 Group and Regional Organization

In the previous five chapters findings have been presented from projects undertaken with a number of particular kinds of hospital staff. In this chapter we shall present the outcomes of certain projects concerned with broader organizational issues, and so step forward to look at group and regional organization as a whole. Specifically, we shall consider findings from project-work on the subjects of:

(1) the exact operational functions to be carried out within an existing hospital region, and which of these are at present carried out by the R.H.B. and which by the H.M.C.;

(2) the role that members of H.M.C. are expected to play, and their relation individually and as a group to the R.H.B.;

(3) the real nature of the present relationship of R.H.B. officers to H.M.C. officers.[1]

The questions listed above do not by any means systematically exhaust all the important issues that might be raised in relation to regional organization. The form of this list simply reflects the main issues of larger organization which have so far been explored in the natural development of project work.[2]

Nevertheless when the material presented is added to that of previous chapters, a certain broad picture of present regional

---

[1] Although the explicit framework of discussion here is regional organization, much of the discussion, particularly of the first question, is also relevant to teaching groups under Board of Governors, with certain obvious translations.

[2] A major project on the internal organization of officers at R.H.B. level is currently in hand but for reasons of confidentiality one cannot at the time of writing report on it.

organization begins to emerge, and this is described towards the end of the chapter. Again, as for so many of the other subjects considered, the general focus lies somewhere between the extant and the requisite. In some sense the picture can claim to mirror the reality of present hospital organization. At the same time it would be idle to pretend that this view was already generally recognized, understood, and accepted. In most places where project-work was undertaken there was no one precise view of organization to be had, either implicit in assumption or explicit in statement. And of course, in the process of clarification the stress has been on describing not just what is, but what ought to be in order to facilitate work and personal relationship. Generally the status of the result might be fairly described as an attempt to formulate the sort of organization that either is in operation and regarded as broadly satisfactory, or might readily be brought into operation within the present main forms and constraints of the service. In this it is in keeping with the title of this Part of the book – Patterns of Existing Hospital Organizations – and distinguishable from formulations in the next Part, which consider more radical alternatives.

Finally, although the picture obtained is one of an organization about to undergo the most fundamental transformation,[3] much of the information has longer-term value as it reveals situations and factors which are likely to be of relevance in any foreseeable service of the future. Consideration of the detailed aims of the present Hospital Service, for example, paves the way to a possible statement of the detailed aims of an integrated health service; the problems that members of present H.M.C.s experience in perceiving appropriate roles for themselves may well have equal relevance to members of the governing bodies of new authorities; and it is very likely that the views of H.M.C. and R.H.B. officers on their mutual relationships will be directly transferable to the mutual relationships of officers at successive tiers in the new service.

The Operational Activities of the Hospital Service

Over the course of several years' work in regions and teaching groups, we have returned increasingly to the question of definition

[3] In the projected re-organization of the National Health Service, following legislation, in 1974.

of *operational activities* even though this question has never at any stage been explicitly posed as a separate project for study.[4] The reason for this preoccupation is simply that as more and more details of the organization of various parts of the service came into view, it becomes increasingly essential to have some fundamental frame of reference by which to orient them. We are using operational functions or activities here as defined in Chapter 3 – those which directly satisfy the specific objects of the organization concerned.

Until some explicit statement has been made of what activities the hospital service is in existence to carry out, it is impossible to get a coherent view of the nature of the present organization, or to consider any substantial questions of what constitutes good or bad organization, or good or bad management, in the service. Organizational forms and management practices only acquire significance and value in relation to the ends for which they are employed.[5] Also, as we have said, consideration of a statement of present aims facilitates the production of a statement of possible aims for a reorganized and integrated health service.

The principal objects of the present Hospital Service are, in the words of the N.H.S. Act 1946: 'to provide ... hospital accommodation, medical, nursing or other services required at or for the purpose of hospitals ... the service of specialists....' (Section 3); and later, through the medium of teaching hospitals: 'to provide for the university with which the hospital is associated ... facilities ... for clinical teaching and research' (Section 12). A possible rendering of these general objects into a more specific set of operational activities to be carried out has evolved from project-discussion, and is shown in Table 10·1.

---

[4] The question has however for some time been recognized as an important one, by those with whom we work, and it has received much discussion in conferences, and more recently, within the Project Steering Committee of the North West Metropolitan Regional Hospital Board. On the recommendation of the latter body the Board itself have now approved in principle a statement of operational activities essentially the same as that shown in Figure 10·1 below.

[5] This is not to suggest that organizational goals are the only *determinants* of requisite organization. As was recognized in Chapter 4 requisite organization will depend as well on a variety of environmental, technological, and social, factors, as well as the objects to be achieved.

Table 10.1   The Operational Activities of the Hospital Service

The provision, integration and development of

1. (Certain Aspects of) Preventive Medicine:
    1.1 health education,
    1.2 health screening – e.g. mass X-ray, quarantine facilities for airports, cervical smears;
2. (Certain Aspects of Primary Care – i.e. primary diagnosis and immediate treatment;
    2.1 accident and emergency services;
3. Specialist Care or Advice – i.e. treatment or advice in the hospital (or sometimes in the home) by specialists to whom cases are referred:
    3.1 by medically-qualified specialists, in for example surgery, anaesthetics, physical medicine, psychiatry, radiology, etc., etc.
    3.2 by paramedical specialists, in for example, pharmacy, physiotherapy, medical physics, dietetics, psychiatric social work, etc., etc.
4. Nursing and Midwifery – in the hospital;
5. Basic Hospital Facilities – for the patients of medical specialists *and* of general practitioners;
    5.1 admission and discharge facilities;
    5.2 ward, clinic and theatre facilities (including accommodation and meals;
    5.3 miscellaneous site facilities (e.g. car parks, telephones, shops);
    5.4 facilities for the compulsory detention of psychiatric patients;
6. Facilities for Clinical Teaching and Research;
7. Training for nurses and paramedical workers.

The list is essentially a list of *services* to be provided – the majority to patients, but some by way of research facilities and training services for present and future members of the health professions. Implicit in any value-statement of services desired, however, are two other value-statements:

(i) that the services shall be in a continual state of development so as to meet the changing needs of the service-receivers through the passage of time as effectively and efficiently as possible (e.g. that clinical services shall be expanded or reduced according to changing patterns of disease in the community); and
(ii) that each service shall be integrated as well as possible with any

other that the same service-receivers may need (e.g. that services from midwives, general practitioners, and specialist obstetricians, shall be fully co-ordinated in any particular maternity case).

In other words the development of services and their integration with each other (and for that matter with the services of any complementary authorities) is part and parcel of operational work.

Coming to the list itself, it will be obvious that some of the activities included are basic to any hospital: the very word 'hospital' implies the presence of ward facilities, admission and discharge facilities, and the provision of nursing, as well as the availability of the service of doctors, whether specialists or general practitioners.[6] Other operational activities such as the provision of nurse training schools, on the other hand, need not be provided in every hospital, but must be provided for somewhere within the service.

To start at the beginning of the health-activity cycle, there are of course certain aspects of preventive medicine (Item 1) that the current hospital service is under obligation to engage in. Certain health-screening activities, for example, the taking of cervical smears, or the carrying out of mass chest X-rays are, or have been, well established. Over and above this, many people in the service feel that the position of health education for the general public must be included as a prime function, although the location of accountability in the present structure for pursuing this activity is not altogether clear.

The distinction between Item 2 (Provision of Primary Care) and Item 3 (Provision of Specialist Care or Advice) is essentially between those sources of clinical services to which a patient may refer himself, and those to which he must be referred by a general practitioner, or by another specialist. Given this distinction, only the accident and emergency services of hospitals fall within the primary care category.

On the other hand, practically the whole of the provision of

---

[6] It is necessary here to correct any over-emphasis on medical treatment alone in considering in total what constitutes a hospital. As Rosen (1963) points out, at earlier periods of history the hospital did not necessarily even provide medical attention. In medieval times the hospital 'remained a combination of an institution for the care of the sick, an old-age home, an almshouse, and an orphanage, possibly a guesthouse' (p. 15). 'Illness creates dependency. The sick need not only medical treatment, but also personal care and shelter' (p. 1).

specialist services rests with the present hospital services (which is of course more strictly referred to as 'hospital and specialist' service – see N.H.S. Act 1946).

Item 4 (Provision of Nursing and Midwifery) refers here to the *characteristic* services that nurses and midwives provide – basic nursing care, the obstetric work of midwives, and the administration of prescribed medical treatment and basic nursing care by nurses and midwives. It does not include the ancillary domestic activities which many nurses in fact perform, or their activities as general co-ordinators of service or 'site-managers', for example, at ward-level.

Item 5 (Basic Hospital Facilities) refers strictly to facilities for patients. The availability of skilled nurses, doctors and other specialists does not in itself make a hospital. It must be supplemented by the facilities of accommodation and equipment of a specialized kind, by meals, by services to help the admission and discharge of patients, and ideally by a number of other miscellaneous facilities for patients.

Item 6 (Provision of Facilities for Clinical Research and Teaching) applies most specifically though not exclusively to teaching hospitals. Here are hospitals whose operational activities include not only the normal care of patients, but also, and quite fundamentally, the provision of facilities for research and for the training of medical undergraduates and postgraduates.

It is perhaps arguable whether Item 7 (Training for Nurses and Paramedical Workers) should be included in the operational list. Certainly there does not appear to be any explicit duty to provide such training laid down in legislation. The fundamental question is whether the hospital service is required as an 'output' independent of its other needs, to produce a continuing supply of trained nurses and paramedical workers; if so the work is operational.

Distinction between Operational and Other (Non-Operational) Activities

Of course, many other activities must be performed if the hospital service is to maintain and improve itself. Buildings must be put up and maintained, staff recruited and paid, materials and equipment purchased, staff hostels provided, linen cleaned, accounting and statistical records kept, and so on. These are the other, or non-operational activities. As discussed in Chapter 3, they are no less essential than operational activities, but they are secondary or subsidiary in status.

The criterion for deciding whether an activity, for example, nurse training, is operational, is whether it is an end in itself. If it is a means to some other organizational end, it is non-operational. Thus, the provision of an admissions and bookings service (usually or mainly the responsibility of a 'medical records' department) although it has elements of means-to-a-treatment-end about it, also stands as a service in its own right. One can readily imagine patients complimenting a hospital on the quality of its reception service, in their minds, whilst separately assessing the quality of nursing and medical services they receive thereafter. The ultimate test of whether an activity is operational is whether those who establish, sanction and finance the service (in this case Parliament) agree that any activity is an 'end' or 'output' for the service. If the hospital service is obliged (to return to the earlier example) to produce a steady supply of trained nurses, over and above its own internal needs, then that work is operational; otherwise not.

The *significance* of the specification of operational, as distinct from non-operational, activities is threefold. First of all, as has been pointed out, unless some statement or understanding of operational activity exists, there can be no logical basis for starting in the first place to organize and recruit staff.[7] Secondly there can be no systematic attempt to monitor and evaluate the effectiveness and efficiency of the service as a whole, though the relative *weightings* given to achievements in different operational areas are another matter. Thirdly, it seems likely that organizational relationships of different kinds are characteristic of roles according to whether they are operational or non-operational. For example, collateral and treatment-prescribing types are characteristic of relationships between operational roles; whilst non-operational roles are characteristically staff-officer or service-giving in type. Thus the clarifica-

---

[7] Oddly enough, it is easier to make assumptions about the non-operational activities required to be carried out in any organization, than (in the absence of any other information) to make assumptions about the operational activity. It is fair to assume that any organization will need, for example, to recruit staff, to purchase equipment, and to maintain records of expenditure. The distinctive character of any specific organization rests in the definition of its operational activities, and this cannot be guessed until the founders or sponsors give appropriate indications.

tion of the operational/non-operational distinction may pave the way to discovering or recognizing the appropriate organizational roles for people to play.

The Present Distribution within the Region of Accountability for Performance of Operational Activities

The great majority of the operational activities listed above are actually performed at H.M.C. level rather than at Regional level. Broadly the H.M.C. is currently the prime operational authority, whilst the R.H.B. maintains a supportive and directive role in carrying out such non-operational activities as:

(1) planning and carrying through all major building projects, though minor projects are carried out by the H.M.C.s themselves;
(2) providing certain centralized supporting services – training, supplies, management services;
(3) exerting a general control of establishments, organization, and training;
(4) exerting a general control of financial expenditure;
(5) monitoring standards of operational performance and taking action to maintain and improve them.

However, the R.H.B. does itself carry out certain minor operational activities in the health screening field (Item (1) above) – for example, mass radiography. More importantly, as it is directly concerned in the negotiation of contracts of employment for consultants and certain other senior medical staff, to this extent it is also directly concerned with the provision of specialist care and advice (Item (3) above). As was discussed in Chapter 5, consultants are accountable only to their employing authority itself, and then only in particular respects. Moreover (as discussed in Chapter 5 and 6) they are often in full-managerial control of considerable numbers of paramedical staff, in addition to junior medical staff. If consultants are accountable only to the R.H.B., then it must follow that the R.H.B. is in a real sense accountable in turn for the substantial specialist services controlled by consultants. At the same time, the H.M.C. undoubtedly has a role to play in monitoring, co-ordinating, and supporting, the activities of all hospital doctors and paramedical staff subordinate to them who work in their hospitals. Over and above this, one could argue that the R.H.B.'s function of planning the provision of medical and hospital facilities throughout the Region, integrally linked as it is with the development of operational services, is a further operational activity itself.[8]

At hospital level itself the main providers of operational services are:

(1) *doctors* (or *specialized dentists*) in providing specialist medical care and advice, such preventive medicine as is carried out, and accident and emergency services;

(2) *paramedical staff*, in providing specialist paramedical care and advice, and training for students;

(3) *nurses and midwives*, in providing specific nursing and midwifery care, training for learner-nurses and midwives, certain admission and discharge services, and certain ward, clinic, and theatre, facilities (e.g. arranging for visits of district nurses following discharge, monitoring supplies of medical and surgical items in clinics and theatres);

(4) *certain other staff who give services directly to patients* (e.g. receptionists, medical secretaries, ward housekeepers, theatre attendants, and caterers) in providing or helping to provide various admission and discharge facilities, ward clinic and theatre facilities for the compulsory detention of psychiatric patients.[9]

By contrast, engineers, builders, cleaners, laundry workers, supplies staff, finance and (most) clerical staff, lay administrators, nursing administration and certain others, do not give services directly to patients, or directly provide any of the other services listed above as operational, and are therefore 'non-operational' – though, as mentioned before, not necessarily thereby any less essential.

The Role of the H.M.C.

Although H.M.C.s are to disappear in the forthcoming reorganization of the Health Service, certain findings from project-work we have carried out with H.M.C. members, have longer-term interest since they bear on general questions such as:

(a) the appropriate role for individuals from various backgrounds

[9] It is not currently clear who at hospital level is accountable for the remaining operational activity listed in Fig. 10·1 – the provision of facilities for clinical teaching and research.

[8] See Chapter 3, Note 7, for a discussion of the conceptual issue involved here.

who are appointed to be members of governing bodies of public authorities; and

(b) the exact quality of organizational relationships between appointed authorities and subordinate authorities in a national service.

Let us start with some factual details about the composition of H.M.C.s. All members of H.M.C.s are appointed by their R.H.B. following consultations with appropriate local interest groups.[10] It is worthy of note that the role of chairman is filled, not by election from amongst members as is normal committee procedure, but by specific appointment by the R.H.B. The final composition to be attained is not specified in legislation, but in addition to those elected purely on individual merit there will usually be members associated with each of the following interests:

(1) elected local authorities;
(2) voluntary bodies concerned with hospital work;
(3) consultant staff;[11]
(4) general practitioners in the catchment area of the hospital;[11]
(5) local Health and Welfare departments;[11]
(6) nursing (hospital or community);
(7) local industry and commerce;
(8) (on occasion) other bodies, e.g. trade unions.

How exactly do H.M.C. members see their roles in practice? Project-work with fourteen members of one H.M.C., including the chairman, produced the following agreed conclusions, after a number of discussions with individuals and the group as a whole.

In the first round of discussions a strong impression was received that whilst it was acknowledged that the R.H.B. were in an authoritative position (and particularly in respect of the chairman, who was regarded by some other members as having a special intermediary function between the R.H.B. and the H.M.C.) individual members nevertheless had separate and major duties, independently of the R.H.B., to represent other groups, such as the patient, the local community, staff of the hospital and so on.[12] For example,

---

[10] See N.H.S. Act 1946, 3rd Schedule.

[11] Total medical membership is limited to 25% of the whole.

[12] This view is apparently not restricted to members of this particular H.M.C. An authoritative guide issued by the Institute of Hospital (now Health Service) Administrators (Stuart-Clark, 1956) on the work of the management committee member states that the responsibility of the H.M.C.

were an H.M.C. member who was also a local councillor to receive a complaint direct from some constituent of his who reckoned that he had received poor treatment in some way at the hospital, a feeling would readily emerge of its being this member's special role in these circumstances to see that 'they' (the hospital authorities, officers, doctors, etc.) gave a proper account of the matter up to the point where he, and his constituent if possible, were reasonably satisfied. Again, where a doctor from the hospital was also a member of the H.M.C. it would be (and often was) seductively easy to regard himself as specially qualified to speak for his medical colleagues when some matter – say visiting hours for patients – came up for discussion, on which a medical view was desired. Feelings like this were reinforced by the perceived composition of the H.M.C., which apparently included 'representatives' of local authority, medical staff, nursing, and so on.

Obviously all turned on exactly what was meant by 'representative'. As analysis of this question went on in discussions a new view gradually emerged, with new implications for behaviour and perhaps, indeed, for organizational structure. A statement was finally agreed by members of the H.M.C., from which the following extracts are drawn:

The Meaning of 'Representative'

Representatives arise where a group of people (e.g. doctors, patients, staff) or an organization (e.g. the local health department) want to have a spokesman who will put forward their views, and perhaps negotiate as well on their behalf.

For satisfactory representation two things are necessary:
– the group or organization concerned must be able to choose their own representative in the first place (this means in practice a

---

member 'is first and foremost to the patient, whose representative in a sense he is' (p.11). The Report of the Ely Committee of Inquiry (1969), who were concerned with the performance of an apparently inadequate H.M.C., serves only to further the role-confusion of the poor H.M.C. member: 'An H.M.C. (or other hospital authority) has ... several conflicting responsibilities. As the representative of the consumer it must see that complaints are brought forward and investigated. As an employer it must see that its staff are protected from unjust attack. As manager and purveyor of a service it must make appropriate management decisions in light of a complaint – and at the same time defend itself against unjust attack. And it must discharge, and appear to discharge, all these functions with a proper sense of justice.' (Para. 469).

process of election where a group is concerned, or appointment where an organization is concerned);
– the group or organization must be able to change their representative if they do not find his performance satisfactory.

Are H.M.C. Members Representatives?
In this sense, it is evident that neither the H.M.C. as a whole, nor individual members, are representative of any particular group (other than the R.H.B.) as it is presently constituted. More specifically:
– 'lay' members of the H.M.C. (whether nominated by local authorities, by voluntary bodies associated with the hospital, or from some other source) are not representatives of the general public or the consumer;
– medical members are not representatives of medical staff;
– officers of the local authority do not represent the local health department;
– general practitioners are not representatives of their colleagues in the catchment area of the hospital

From this it follows that the members are not authorized to press the needs of a single interest group over and above the general requirements of the hospital as a whole, as laid down in broad policy terms by the R.H.B.

Having said this, it is certainly part of the job of H.M.C. members to have concern for the needs of patients and staff, and to take into account the views of the other relevant groups. Far from being inconsistent with the role of the H.M.C. as R.H.B. subordinate, this is an essential component of it.

From this point, real representatives of these various groups, where they existed, were readily identified in discussion – the chairman of the Medical Staff Committee for consultants, the chairman of the Local Medical Committee for general practitioners, the local council for the local community. However, it was recognized that whereas chief officers attended H.M.C. meetings and could and would communicate hospital staff opinion, no genuine elected representative existed for groups of hospital staff other than doctors in this particular Hospital Group.[13]

If the view of the consultants on visiting, or on priorities for redevelopment of wards or any other issue were required, then

[13] Some staff were however represented through trade union officials, and at a later stage, a joint consultative committee involving elected staff representatives was resuscitated in this particular Group.

surely (given the inability to communicate with forty or fifty at once) it would be better to talk with their duly-elected representative. If it were requisite to know what the community as a whole thought about some proposed closure of a small geriatric hospital, then it might be appropriate to ascertain the views of their representatives, the local authority, approaching through officers of that authority in the first instance (e.g. the clerk to the authority, the Medical Officer of Health or the Director of Social Services).

In relation to complaints and grievances the role of H.M.C. members again appeared in a different light following discussion and analysis.

At an early stage in discussion a suggestion arose that H.M.C. members, jointly or severally, might have some special role to play in respect of complaints by patients (for example where a patient privately approached an individual H.M.C. member) or staff grievances (for example where a junior staff member relayed a grievance to an H.M.C. member during the course of a hospital visit). The H.M.C. member in this situation might perhaps be conceived as playing some independent or 'ombudsman'-type role. Later discussion suggested, however, that the concern of H.M.C. members with problems of individual patients and grievances of staff was again wholly consistent with their role as ultimate managers of the hospital, subject to the R.H.B. Such problems would normally be relayed by the H.M.C. member concerned to the appropriate hospital officers to deal with them in the first instance. At a later stage, the H.M.C. as a body might be involved in either these same complaints of patients or grievances of staff, as they worked their way up the management hierarchy in accordance with existing procedure.

The members of this H.M.C., then, recognized themselves clearly in the end as members of a body subordinate in a general sense to the R.H.B. and accountable to the R.H.B. and to the R.H.B. only. But was the relationship between the R.H.B. and the H.M.C. exactly a superior-subordinate one? Looking at the exact definition evolved in the research (see Chapter 4) the central elements of authority in a full superior-subordinate or managerial relationship are:

(1) the right to prescribe work and assign tasks;
(2) the right to have (at least) veto over appointment;
(3) the right to assess, and reward or sanction;
(4) the right to be able to initiate transfer or dismissal.

Clearly the R.H.B. had control over appointment of H.M.C. members, individually and in aggregate. The right to dismiss individual members, on the other hand, would only effectively be deployed at the time when a member's period of service came up for termination or renewal. Apart from this, no other formalized sanctions existed – for example, it was not conceivable to think of personal assessment records being maintained in respect of individual members, as could be and often are maintained for serving officers. Finally, and most difficult of all, could the R.H.B. prescribe work and set tasks for the H.M.C. in all or any aspects of their activities, as a superior could for his subordinate?

Now this has been a well-recognized and controversial question since the establishment of the Health Service. (See note at end of chapter.) The trouble is that two separate issues are almost always confused in discussions. The first is whether the R.H.B. has *rights* to direct H.M.C.s should it wish, in various matters, and if so, whether or not there is any limit to the matters in which it may so direct. The second (which only arises if the R.H.B. do have rights of direction), is the extent to which it is *desirable* for the R.H.B. to exercise their rights in any given case; or put another way, the extent to which the R.H.B. should allow H.M.C.s freedom to act at their own discretion. The same question arises in fact in even the most straightforward relation between superior and subordinate. Even granted that the superior has the right to prescribe the work of his subordinate in any authorized respect, he has still to decide when to intervene and when to leave alone. If he delegates too much, he runs the risk that the subordinate will for one reason or another misuse his freedom. If he arrogates all decisions to himself, then he literally does all the work, and his subordinate becomes redundant. Much of course turns on the assessed capacity of the subordinate in this situation.

In discussion with senior officers from one R.H.B., the H.M.C. members in the project mentioned above, and senior officers from this and many other Hospital Groups, whenever the analysis has been pursued to its conclusion it appears to have been accepted that the R.H.B. have ultimate rights (within the prescriptions of central government) to prescribe to the H.M.C. in any matters on which the latter might themselves act.[14] In other words, it is

---

[14] But see further thoughts on this matter in Chapter 13.

generally accepted that H.M.C.s in the end have no inalienable rights or powers of their own, in spite of their independent legal existence. At the same time, it has also become evident in these discussions that this analysis of the situation is not necessarily universally recognized or acted upon in practice (or has not been in the past) within the particular Region concerned.

Nevertheless, even supposing this full prescriptive authority is granted, there are the other reasons stated why this relationship could not exactly be described as a superior-subordinate one. It is no doubt of the same family as a superior-subordinate one, but arising as it does between group and group, rather than individual and individual, with the different social consequences this inevitably brings, it probably warrants a separate description and title, as suggested in Chapter 4.

Relation of R.H.B. Officers to the H.M.C.

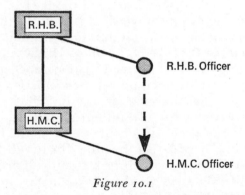

Figure 10.1

Given this authoritative relationship between R.H.B. as a corporate body and H.M.C., what does this imply for the relationship of the R.H.B. officer to the H.M.C. and its staff? Primarily the relationship will be one between officer and officer, and normally between officers concerned with the same specialty e.g. Regional Nursing Officer and Chief Nursing Officer, Regional Engineer and Group Engineer, Regional Treasurer and Group Treasurer.

Manifestly, regional officers have no authority in their own right over their group colleagues, being servants of entities which are legally distinct and separate. The first loose formulation often posed in project discussions of this relationship is that the regional officer has purely an 'advisory' relationship to his counterpart at group. Now if this were really the case, firstly there would presumably be no contact between the two unless initiated by the group officer, and secondly, any comments or suggestions made by the regional officer following the initiative of the group officer could be taken or ignored by the latter, as he judged fit. But neither of these is the case. Regional officers regularly take the initiative in approaching group colleagues, and what they say on many occasions quite certainly has a stronger flavour than mere 'advice'. If the Region are introducing a computer to handle all accounts, the way in which basic financial data must be prepared and fed to the computer by Group Treasurers is a matter for instruction by the Regional Treasurer, not advice. Nor is the Regional Engineer's comment on the technical desirability of a particular scheme for providing standby power supplies costing many thousands of pounds 'advisory'. Nor is the Regional Nursing Officer's views on the appropriate number and grades of nursing management establishment in a pilot 'Salmon' reorganization approved by the Region 'advisory'. Examples could be multiplied indefinitely.

In fact project discussions have produced the following formulation[15] which, preliminary though it may be, is no doubt an advance on the unrealistic notion of a simple 'advisory' relationship.

The relationship between an R.H.B. officer and his H.M.C. counterpart (e.g. Regional Treasurer and Group Treasurer, Regional Nursing officer and Chief Nursing Officer of the Group) is not a superior-subordinate one, but does involve authority, and has extantly the following characteristics:

- The R.H.B. officer provides advice on request for his H.M.C counterpart, on any subject within their common field.
- The R.H.B. officer monitors the adherence of the H.M.C. and its officers to R.H.B. policies within his given field; that is, he checks on actual activities, discusses and negotiates changes with his H.M.C. counterpart where necessary, and reports on results to the R.H.B.
- In many cases, he participates in the selection of his H.M.C. counterpart (for example, in the case of nursing the R.N.O. takes part in the selection of C.N.O.s).

[15] The formulation was agreed in the first instance with the chief officers of one H.M.C. group, and subsequently by a number of regional officers on the Project Steering Committee of the Region concerned.

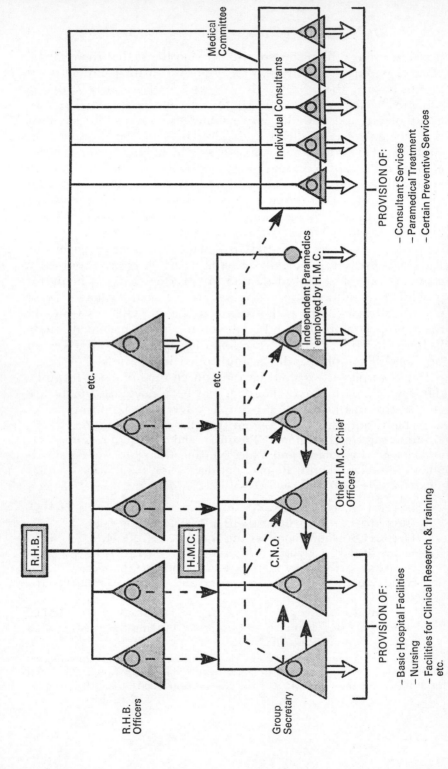

Figure 10.2 A 'Multi-partite Management' Model of Group Organization

The 'policies' referred to here can relate to any aspect of the field concerned: to techniques, procedures, organization, establishment, recruitment, and training.

In discussing the interpretation of R.H.B. policy with the H.M.C. officer, the R.H.B. officer carries prescriptive authority. The R.H.B. officer can insist on a certain interpretation of policy, following discussion, which is then binding on his H.M.C. counterpart, unless the latter indicates that he wishes it to be referred to the H.M.C., for ultimate testing with the R.H.B. (In practice, a discussion between R.H.B. and H.M.C. in such a situation would usually be undertaken by the respective chairmen.)

As it stands, this is the 'functional monitoring and co-ordinating relationship' defined in Chapter 4, differing from 'attachment' chiefly by lack of (at any rate) explicit authority to veto selection in all cases, to join in formal assessment of personal capability, and to initiate transfer or dismissal.

A General Picture of Present Regional Organization

It is now possible to bring together the project-findings reported in this chapter and previous ones, so as to produce a general picture

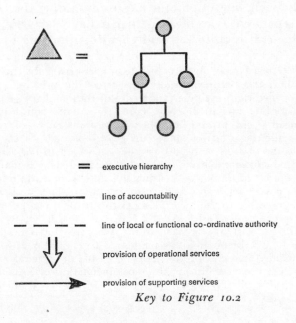

= executive hierarchy

———————— line of accountability

— — — — line of local or functional co-ordinative authority

⇓ provision of operational services

——————▶ provision of supporting services

Key to Figure 10.2

of regional organization which fills in, as it were, the main factual outlines taken as a starting-point in Chapter 2. Figure 10.2 shows typical organization of an H.M.C. group in relation to the R.H.B. and its officers, as it appears following analysis and clarification. It shows the main role-structures and the disposition of operational work amongst them.

Conventional wisdom has it that the management structure at H.M.C. level is tri-partite in nature, a troika of chief administrator, Chief Nursing Officer and hospital doctors (through the person of the most senior medical man in official position).[16] In fact, the reality might more aptly be described as 'multi-partite'. For one thing, as we have seen there are a number of senior officers at group level who are generally (though by no means universally) regarded as accountable directly to the governing body, not only the Group Secretary and the Chief Nursing Officer[17] but also the Treasurer and perhaps the Engineer, Building Supervisor, the Chief Pharmacist and a number of other heads of paramedical departments. For another, as we have seen consultants are *not* organized hierarchically under one medical director or chairman. Each is in effect his own departmental head, some with very considerable establishments of junior medical and paramedical staff.

As we have also seen, one important means of binding the work of these various separate hierarchies together in day by day activity is through the general monitoring and co-ordinating role of the

[16] The Bradbeer Report (1954), an early and major report on the internal administration of hospitals, enthusiastically supported the principal of a triple partnership of medical, nursing and lay administration (Paras. 20, 21) though the general notion was an old one (Para. 18). At the same time it did recognize the need at group level for 'one chief administrative officer ... with a general co-ordinating function under the governing body' (Para. 22).

[17] The position of the matron or head nurse has according to the Salmon Report (1966) suffered considerable vicissitudes (Para. 2). Although matrons in the voluntary hospitals of Florence Nightingale's time were made responsible directly to the governing body, those in local authority hospitals were more likely to be responsible to the medical superintendent in charge. With the creation of hospital groups following the National Health Service, the absence of a group nursing role weakened the voice of nursing at the highest levels, whilst in Scotland matrons tended to be subordinate to the medical superintendent commonly in post. However with the general establishment of group chief nurses following the recommendation of Salmon to appoint such 'responsible directly to the governing body' (Para. 6.38) there was a rise in status again.

chief administrator – the Group Secretary. Another important means on the medical side – appropriate to the natural collegiate structure of medical consultants – is through medical committees with self-elected chairmen. As was pointed out in Chapter 5, the elected representative post of Chairman of Medical Committee should be rigorously distinguished from that of medical administrator (under whatever name) appointed by the governing body. Where posts of the latter kind exist project-work (albeit limited) suggests that they too will be directly accountable to the governing body.[18]

Finally, we have a strong suggestion from one project at any rate, that members of the H.M.C. itself are accountable as a body to the R.H.B., and subject to the direction of the latter in all matters in which the R.H.B. itself has authority. Individual members of H.M.C.s have no role as representatives of particular interest-groups, but are appointed to give the benefit of their particular contributions as individuals from a variety of backgrounds, in what should be a true committee-decision-making process. 'True' representatives of various interest-groups are to be discerned separately: members of local authorities, members of Local Medical Committees, and (for hospital staff) members of medical staff committees, and in some cases, joint consultative councils.

Note to Chapter 10

Control of R.H.B.s over H.M.C.s (page 201)

The original N.H.S. Act (1946) clearly stated that the R.H.B.s had powers of direction over H.M.C.s (as did the Minister over R.H.B.s). It shall be the duty of the Hospital Management Committee of any hospital or group of hospitals, *subject to and in accordance*

---

[18] The Ely Report (1959) and the Farleigh Report (1970) – both reports of inquiry into malfunctioning hospitals – found evidence of great lack of clarity as to where the roles of senior administrator and medical superintendent began and ended and how they fitted together (Ely Para. 386, Farleigh Para. 76). On the other hand, in two cases of medical administrator roles come across in our project-work (one a medical superintendent in a psychiatric group, the other a medical administrator, by this name, in a general group) both were seen as subsidiary to the chief administrator as far as the general co-ordination of the work of the hospitals in the group was concerned.

with regulations and such directions as may be given by the
Minister or the Regional Hospital Board, to control and manage
that hospital or group of hospitals on behalf of the Board, and for
that purpose to exercise on behalf of the Board such functions of
the Board relating to that hospital or group of hospitals as may
be prescribed. (Section 12 (2) – our italics.)

However early Departmental Circulars (R.H.B. (47) 1 and H.M.C.
(48) 1) emphasized that H.M.C.s were to be given considerable freedom to get on with their own business. The Guillebaud Committee
(1956) after reviewing the shifts on opinion on this question since
the establishment of the N.H.S. themselves concluded:

that R.H.B.s should be told and H.M.C.s should accept that the
Regional Boards are responsible for exercising a general oversight
and supervision over the administration of the hospital service in
their Regions. It is a corollary of this recommendation that the
Ministry should leave the task of supervising the H.M.C.s to the
Regional Boards, and should not itself undertake this task over
the head of the Boards. (Para. 212.)

Nevertheless considerable doubt still reigned, as we evidenced for
example by the Committee of Inquiry into the disturbing situation
at the Ely Hospital for subnormal patients.

Standards of performance thus clearly need to be checked from
time to time by somebody who is not responsible for day-to-day
management of a hospital like Ely. This function has not apparently been discharged within Wales by the R.H.B. It was explained
to us that the Board's officers did not regard themselves as entitled
to perform any inspectorial function of the kind we had in mind.
(Paras. 461-462.)

Following this Report a Departmental Circular was issued to clarify
the relationship of R.H.B.s and H.M.C.s (HM (69) 59) though, with
its air of giving with one hand (Para. 2), only to take back with
another (Para. 3), it is doubtful whether it achieved its object:

2. Regional Hospital Boards carry out their functions as agents
   of the Secretary of State. Hospital Management Committees
   carry out their functions as agents of the Regional Hospital
   Board. Boards and Committees are subject to regulations or
   directions made by the Secretary of State and Committees are
   subject to directions made by Boards.

3. The Secretary of State wishes Hospital Management Committees to exercise their functions without unnecessary intervention by the Regional Hospital Board or by himself.

4. Regional Hospital Boards are however responsible to the
   Secretary of State for the services in their regional areas. He

looks to the Boards to exercise general oversight of the administration and standards of care in the hospital service in their
regions, including whatever arrangements for visiting they
consider appropriate for this purpose.

Nor did Rosemary Stewart's acute and detailed observation of the
response (or in this case, largely non-response) of H.M.C.s to an
important Ministerial Circular on the management of outpatient
departments provide any convincing evidence of the unequivocal
status of the authority of higher echelons in respect of the activities
of H.M.C.s. (See Stewart and Sleeman, 1967.)

Part III

Conclusions and Departures

11 Some General Conclusions from Project-Work So Far

In Part I a number of basic ideas and concepts were described in terms which could be used to analyse and assay organizational structure, and in particular that to be found in hospitals. In Part II were described the results of the use of these basic concepts in the analysis of parts of the existing hospital service, as each became the subject of specific research projects. In this third and final part we shall attempt to discuss some of the main conclusions to be drawn from project-work so far, and to illustrate the implications that they hold for the design of hospitals and health services in general.

In any general and comprehensive consideration of hospital organization at the time of writing it is of course quite impossible to ignore the radical reshaping of the National Health Service which is to come within the next few years. Consequently it is natural to consider the implications of the work done so far not just for hospitals of the future, but for integrated health services as a whole. Indeed at the time of writing members of the project-team are becoming increasingly involved in project-work of precisely this kind.[1] However, this particular book is not primarily about

[1] It has been impossible to ignore larger questions of health service organization too, in conference discussion, so that the material to come has already received some testing within a conference setting with senior officers of the hospital service. The Brunel Hospital Organization Research Unit has recently been asked (1971) by its prime sponsors, the D.H.S.S., to broaden its considerations and its title, from hospitals to health services as a whole. The Unit is already involved in project discussions at D.H.S.S. level on the shape of the new service. At the same time, the work of two sister-units at Brunel – the Social Services Organization Research Unit and the Community Development Project – has also influenced to some degree the thinking in the final part of the book.

the integrated health service of the future, and though the analysis in Part III is extended in many cases to consider likely situations within a future unified national health service, much of the analysis would apply equally to the hospital service as it now exists in Britain, and no doubt in some degree to hospital and health services in many other countries.

Finally, whilst this book can only describe a definite and contained area of work and thinking, and must draw an arbitrary rule across a continuing and expanding process of exploration and analysis, there are of course at any time a number of issues which begin to be distinguished and recognized as significant, but for which neither precise formulation nor specific testing in the conference or the field-project is yet existent. To illustrate the continuing and developing nature of the project-thinking some of these emerging issues are briefly described in Chapter 13.

For a start in this chapter, some general conclusions that can be distilled from the various projects described in Part II will be summarized:

(a) the effects of clinical and professional autonomy and their general implications for organization-structure – the hierarchy ('unified management') and the co-ordinated group ('multi-management');
(b) the general importance of the distinction between ranks and grades in hierarchies, and further implications of this distinction;
(c) the inevitability of 'dual-influence' situations;
(d) the non-representative nature of present statutory bodies.

Clinical and Professional Autonomy

The extreme diversity of occupational or professional groups to be found within the hospital service has been remarked before (Chapter 6). This diversity has no doubt many implications for the coherence and morale of hospital life, but we shall be concerned here chiefly with its implications for organization-structure, and more precisely with implications for the kind of role-relationships that can be established between members of different professional or occupational groups.

For a start, two issues can be distinguished. The first is the general question of professional autonomy and independence, and the second is the more specific question of clinical autonomy, i.e.

autonomy arising directly out of the nature of the doctor- (or therapist-) patient relationship.

The present fact of the clinical autonomy of the medical consultant in hospitals (though not autonomy of other and junior medical grades) was noted in Chapter 5, and its possible exact outlines and content delineated. It was also suggested there that the justification for this autonomy might spring directly from the relationship which in our present society is sought between a patient and the doctor who is responsible for his treatment. If *personalized* treatment, rather than an *agency* treatment is required, then it follows that the physician or therapist must have complete freedom, within certain definite and not readily-alterable limits, to direct that treatment as he thinks fit.

At the same time, if clinical freedom is not to degenerate into clinical licence, society must have some control over the work of the independent therapist; not just over the resources it makes available to him (which it always has) but beyond certain given limits, in the way he uses these resources. In extreme cases where it is plain for all to see, for example, that the doctor concerned is mad, bad, or bone-lazy, there must be effective ways of calling him to account.

If this argument is right, the implications for organizational design in the health field are profound: the work of the doctor (the doctor in charge of the case, that is) can be *monitored* in relation to certain obvious features which might be summarized in the phrase 'conduct and contract', but can neither be *monitored* nor *managed* in relation to the way judgment is exercised within these broad limits. At the most we shall look for mechanisms by which his work may be better co-ordinated with that of his colleagues and of the hospital as a whole, or mechanisms by which his judgment can be subject to the influence without authority of peer-criticism and opinion.[2]

---

[2] In the precise language of the project we shall be looking for *monitoring* relationships, *co-ordinative* relationships and *colleague* or *collegiate* relationships, but not for *managerial* relationships or any of their offshoots (*supervisory* and *staff*). Again, however, it is worth considering Freidson's argument that the quality of medical judgment should be subject to periodic and formal review by some outside body of colleagues, which is linked to possible sanctions, if not to any specific authority to instruct change in practice (Freidson, 1970).

Might other therapeutic occupations too, extantly occupy (or requisitely aspire to) this special position? The evidence from project-work so far is inconclusive. It is perhaps an open question for certain groups of paramedical staff: social workers,[3] dietitians, chiropodists, etc. (see Chapter 6). It is certainly not open for midwives, and other large groups of paramedical staff such as occupational therapists or physiotherapists, who are all subject to medical direction, i.e. working within *treatment-prescribing* relationships.

This brings us to the second issue, broader than clinical autonomy, which is the meaning, if any, to be given to professional autonomy in general. This question arises not only for those occupations which are directly concerned in diagnosis and treatment in individual cases, but also in relation to other groups in the hospital setting such as treasurers or engineers, who lay claim to professional status.

The first and obvious question is what is meant by profession?[4] For the purposes of this discussion it may be sufficient to draw attention to two features of the fully-developed profession:

(1) the existence of at least minimum standards of practice and conduct defined by a distinct professional body and backed by sanctions for non-adherence;
(2) the existence of a body of exclusive knowledge, which is more or less impervious to 'lay' understanding.

The first feature should give rise to few problems, organizationally. It merely needs to be recognized that where such basic and indubitable professional standards exist employed members of that profession, and indeed all other members of the hospital organization, are obliged to observe them.[5] Regardless of what directions they are given by those who have authority over them, treasurers, for example, must observe certain basic proprieties in

[3] There is evidence that social-workers in local authority employment do not carry personalized client responsibility, with associated 'clinical autonomy', but provide together an 'agency-service'. (Rowbottom and Hey, 1970).

[4] See Chapter 5, Note 1.

[5] In the extreme such basic standards merge into more general canons of lawful and proper behaviour, which will be felt to be binding on *all* members of the organization regardless of whether they regard themselves as 'professionals' or not.

the keeping of accounts and handling cash; nurses must observe certain basic proprieties in the treatment of patients; and engineers must observe certain basic rules of safety and good technical practice. Such rules do not preclude the establishment of managerial or any other relationships of 'lay' to 'professional' staff: they merely indicate one of the limits within which managerial authority (if any) could be properly employed. So much then for 'basic' professional standards.

The second issue, what might be called the 'knowledge-gap', raises more difficult problems. Where, or whether, the knowledge-gap between any two occupational-groups in the health field itself precludes the establishment of managerial relationships between a member of one and a member of the other, is still, at the time of writing, very much an open question.

Leaving aside the special question of clinical autonomy discussed above, this more general question turns on what can properly be expected of the superior in a managerial relationship. As discussed in Chapter 6, the question is not whether the manager can *perform* the work of the subordinate but whether he or she could understand it well enough to be able to make general assessments of the all-round ability of the subordinate, to set meaningful tasks, and to help with work-problems. The establishment of co-managerial relationships, 'technical' and 'operational', in an *attachment* situation can be understood as one way of trying to resolve this difficulty.

What has emerged from project-work with some certainty is that what might be called 'professional ranking' operates in this field. The particular issue is not whether members of Profession A can in principle be managed by any others at all outside their professsion, but whether they can be managed in principle by Professions B, C, D, etc. For example, whether nurses could be managed in principle by administrators may be in doubt, but that they could be managed in principle by doctors is in little doubt, even though for various reasons this situation rarely arises in practice in present hospital organization. Whether building staff could be managed by architects or by engineers is one thing: whether they could be managed by administrators (in the particular meaning attached to this term in the health field) is another. In general it may be supposed that where treatment-prescribing is possible, as for example between doctors and many paramedical groups, managerial relationships are also possible in principle.[6]

Implications for Unified- and Multiple-Management Systems

The implications of these matters for the design of hospital organization or any other health service organization are profound. One major concern in any such design-situation will be to establish adequate mechanisms for co-ordination and control. Managerial relationships are powerful means of achieving just this, and also have the effect of concentrating the accountability for the success or failure in few hands, ultimately in one pair where successive layers of managerial relationships are employed.[7] (See Figure 11.1 (a).) However, against this wish for strong control must be offset desires or needs for the establishment of clinical autonomy, and where it is valid, some degree of professional autonomy more generally.

To the extent that these latter requirements are recognized as of paramount importance, there will be a tendency to accept systems in which the binding mechanism is far less than full-managerial, and in fact no more than some kind of monitoring or co-ordinating one. In such a situation, both heads of various professional groups and independent therapists would be accountable directly and only to their employing authorities. Though each head might himself play a full management role in relation to some subordinate hierarchy, the group of heads themselves would not be hierarchically organized: they would be at most a co-ordinated and monitored group. This may be desecribed as a 'multiple-management' situation (Figure 11.1(b)).

Where the heads of hierarchies were doctors or other independent therapists, carrying personal responsibility for their cases, they would not be accountable to the employing authority for the way, within certain basic limits described above, in which they

[6] This is somewhat akin to Freidson's formulation (op cit) of the idea of a 'hierarchy of institutionalized expertise' in which only the highest professions, e.g. medicine, can attain genuine autonomy and 'professional dominance'.

[7] At least one of the motives for reorganization of the National Health Service is just this concentration of accountability and strengthening or establishment of managerial relationships, clearly evidenced for example in the Consultation Document on the Future of the N.H.S. (Department of Health, 1971 – Foreword and Para. 6).

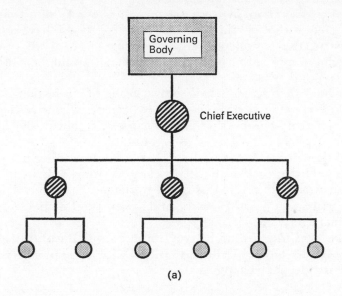

Figure 11.1   Unified and Multiple-Management
(a) *Unified management – the managerial hierarchy*

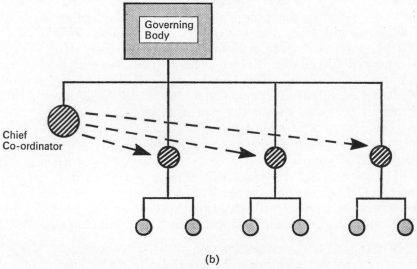

(b) *Multiple management – the Co-ordinated Group*

exercised discretion in carrying out their work, nor would the employing authority, through its governing body, have authority to instruct such independent clinicians. Where they wanted change, the governing body or its officers[8] would be obliged to negotiate and persuade.

On the other hand, where other heads of professional groups were *not* concerned directly with treatment, whatever degree of professional autonomy they might possess, it obviously does not prevent their being regarded as accountable to the governing body for all they do, or (what probably says the same thing better) subject to some degree of authority by the governing body in all aspects of their work. However, this is not to suggest that such a relationship between governing body and chief professional would be fully-managerial in character.

Some possible alternatives of unified- and multi-management structures in more specific situations will be explored in more detail in the next chapter.

Ranks and Grades

Another main finding from project-work so far is the widespread tendency in the present hospital service to confuse what we have here described as the concepts of *rank* (i.e. level in managerial hierarchy) with *grade* (i.e. the status or payment-level of the role). We are here talking of a confusion that arises essentially within managerial hierarchies. Evidence has already been quoted of its occurrence within nursing organization (Chapter 7) and within domestic organization (Chapter 8). Other project-work (not quoted in detail here) has shown that it can arise within administrative organization too, at the 'deputy' and 'assistant' levels, and it is probable that it arises in many other hierarchical situations in larger departments.

The analysis of the situation in nursing presented in Chapter 7 may well stand as a general model here. Not only is executive role confused with grade, but titles (the third factor) are used to refer indiscriminately to each. Titles such as 'senior nursing officer' are

[8] It is significant that it is not felt appropriate to refer to say, medical consultants, as 'officers' of their employing authority. On the other hand this title is easily applicable to many other senior professionals – architects, engineers, treasurers, etc.

made to do duty *both* as indication of grade (and hence salary-range) *and* as indication of the particular range of functions to be carried out, and (implicitly) the nature of role-relationships with associated staff.

As discussed in detail in the same chapter, a number of adverse consequences flow from such confusion. Firstly, it becomes very difficult to conduct a reasoned discussion about the appropriate grading to be attached to any post, since the post cannot be independently identified. Secondly, there is a large danger of assuming that all steps in grade represent full-managerial relationships, thus ignoring the real needs in many situations for supervisory, staff-officer or other co-ordinating, rather than managerial, roles.

Dual-influence situations

Another general finding from the research is of the widespread existence of what have been termed dual-influence situations (Chapter 4), i.e. in general terms, situations in which a member of the service is subject to controls of some kind from two separate points of the organization. Such situations have been discovered, for example, in pharmacy (Chapter 6), in nursing (Chapter 7), in engineering, medical records, supplies, etc. (Chapter 8), and in general, in many situations where staff in one hospital are subject both to local influence and to technical or 'functional' influence from group level. It is also seen at group level, where officers are subject to the dual-influence of their own local administration and of their regional counterparts (Chapter 10). It is, as we have seen, a situation inextricably tied up with the growth of so-called 'functional management'. It must certainly be regarded as an inevitable situation in any large-scale modern organization, and particularly in health organizations, springing as it does from the increasing need for specialist control on the one hand, with the continuing need for local operational co-ordination on the other.

The obvious mistake here would be to think that any one pattern of organizational relationships would do equally for each dual-influence situation. Four different patterns have been spelt out in Chapter 4 – *outposting, attachment or co-management, functional monitoring and co-ordination*, and *secondment*. Perhaps others too are still required. In the next chapter we shall consider further implications of the findings too, for organizational design.

The Non-Representative Nature of Present Statutory Bodies

Finally, one further conclusion bears reiteration, notwithstanding its slender base in actual fieldwork. It is evidently easy to assume that statutory bodies in the present health service, whose members are in fact appointed by higher authorities, either do, or can requisitely, carry out genuine representative functions (Chapter 10). Apart from the harm that such role-confusion might do to the efficient working of such statutory bodies themselves, there is the greater harm done by shielding the real question, which is whether truly-representative bodies of various interest-groups are indeed needed as well, and if so, how they are best established.

In other words what is at issue here is genuine participation, as opposed to the 'mock-democracy'[9] of the present service. Little project-work has as yet been done in this area, but some preliminary thought and analysis are offered in Chapter 13.

[9] We are indebted to our colleague, Professor Maurice Kogan, for this phrase.

12 General Implications for Organizational-Design in the Health Field

In this chapter we shall attempt to show how the findings and conclusions of our project-work so far may be applied to constructing
ranges of possible models for the organization of hospitals and of
health services more generally.

Any sizeable health organization which employs members of a
variety of occupations or professions at a number of widely-spaced
sites, is likely to face certain common problems of co-ordination.

(1) It must somehow effectively co-ordinate the continuing treatment for the individual patient, whenever or wherever it takes
place (as for example, the patient moves from community to
hospital and back) and however many different members of the
service or outside agencies are involved in it (*co-ordination of the
individual case*).

(2) It must effectively co-ordinate the planning and provision of
services as a whole, for whole categories of patients, for example,
for maternity cases, the mentally disordered, or the failing old
(*co-ordination of the 'patient-group'*).

(3) It must effectively co-ordinate the work, training, and development, of particular occupational or professional groups (*occupational co-ordination*).

(4) It must effectively co-ordinate all activities, both operational and
other, carried out by diverse occupations with diverse groups of
patients at any one particular institutional site (*institutional
co-ordination*).

(5) It must effectively co-ordinate the development and provision of
services as a whole, for the authority as a whole (*overall operational co-ordination*).[1]

[1] A similar list has been developed by Naylor (1971), page 18.

There is of course a variety of different possible avenues of attack on these problems, many not directly to do with organizational role-structure. For example, co-ordination may be facilitated by the mere fact of bringing the actors concerned into social proximity: in 'attaching' nurses or social workers to health-centres or to group practices (i.e. of general medical practitioners); or in bringing together hospital doctors, general practitioners and public health (or community) physicians in postgraduate medical centres. It may also be facilitated by fostering more co-operative attitudes through training programmes of various kinds; and so on.

What we can usefully study here, however, is the range of organizational models (i.e. models of role-structure) available, and the likely efficacy of each in promoting co-ordination or otherwise. The remainder of the chapter is devoted to considering just this, in relation to the five fields listed above in which co-ordination is manifestly required.[2]

Models of Organization for the Integrated Treatment of Individual Patients

If one considers the case history of almost any patient who receives hospital treatment, from the moment when he or she in his normal life in the community becomes aware of the need of medical attention to the point when he or she finally returns to that community without need of further aid, one is struck by the variety of people who may be directly concerned with that patient, and the complexity of relationships between them. Consider the not unlikely situation given for example in Figure 12.1(a) in which one case is dealt with at various times by a general practitioner, a medical consultant, his registrar, his houseman; a ward charge nurse, her staff nurse, and a learner nurse; a physiotherapist, a social worker, and a district nurse. Three main varieties of organizational relationships prevail between various actors in this sort of situation:

(a) *hierarchical*, e.g. as between charge nurse and staff nurse, or consultant and registrar;

[2] The thinking here has again been stimulated by a number of discussions with Maurice Naylor, Secretary to the Sheffield Regional Hospital Board, who was currently undertaking research and study in the same field. Although the final formulations are not exactly his (Naylor, 1971) they owe much to his influence.

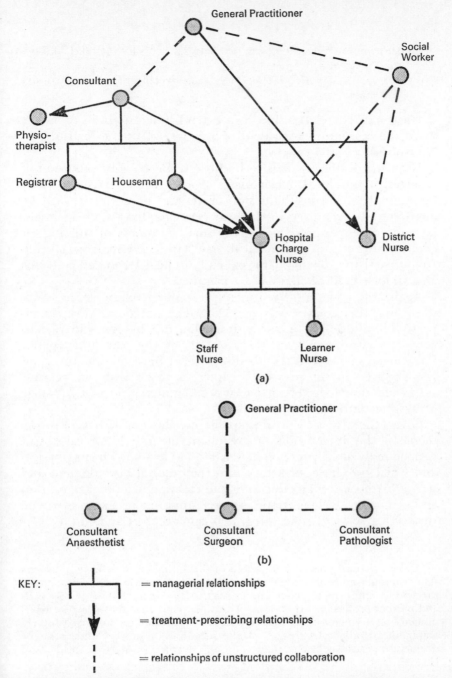

KEY:

    = managerial relationships

    = treatment-prescribing relationships

    = relationships of unstructured collaboration

*Figure 12.1 Examples of Models of Organization for Integrated
Treatment of Individual Cases*

(b) *treatment-prescribing*, e.g. as between consultant and physiotherapist; and,

(c) *unstructured collaboration*, e.g. as between general practitioner
and consultant.

Unstructured relationships can extend indefinitely in each case
when the opinion or treatment of a variety of further consultants
is involved (Figure 12.1(b)).

In principle there seems to be little scope for any extension of
stronger, hierarchical, mechanisms of integration. It is not likely
for example that consultant staff or general practitioners will be
appropriately organized in this way (see Chapter 5). There might
be some opportunities for placing small numbers of nursing, or
certain categories of paramedical, staff within the managerial control of particular doctors – for example in health centres; but such
alterations would be likely to be marginal.

Again, the placing of treatment-prescribing relationships is not
something that could easily be changed or extended. Treatment-
prescribing authority is not a thing that can be given to various
actors or withdrawn from them at will by the particular agency
for whom they work; it is embedded deeper in social structure, and
(as suggested in the previous chapter) is to do with the relative
status and knowledge of particular occupational groups at any stage
of social evolution.

Given these facts, the inescapable conclusion is that improvement in the integration of treatment of individual cases will
depend most heavily on non-organizational factors: on the physical
and social proximity of actors, and the gradual development and
strengthening through education and training of a particular ethos
and custom of co-operation,[3] or the provision of more adequate
supporting services (like integrated case records) and so on.

[3] It is particularly true of the professional training or 'socialization' process
that it imbues not only specialist knowledge and skill, but also enumerable
precepts of appropriate behaviour in relation to clients, fellow-professionals
and partner-professions. It is probably at this point that the strongest determinants of co-operative or non-co-operative attitudes are laid. See for example the detailed description of the socialization process undergone by
doctors during the course of their training presented in Merton, Reader and
Kendall (1957).

Models of Organization for the Integrated Provision and Development of Services for a Category of Cases

Turning from treatment in the individual case to planning of the service as a whole for particular categories of cases (for example, maternity cases, psychiatric cases, or geriatric cases) the scope for alternative or new organizational models seems more open.

For a start, however, very large numbers of people are likely to be concerned with services for any given class of patients in the locality of any health authority. If for example services for psychiatric patients are considered (see Figure 12.2) at least the following will be directly concerned:

- all the general practitioners
- all the specialists in psychiatry, both junior and senior
- all nurses from psychiatric wards
- all occupational therapists who work with psychiatric patients
- all the administrators or executive officers concerned with general administration of institutions dealing with psychiatric cases
- all social workers within hospitals who work with psychiatric patients
- all the fieldwork-staff, and a proportion of the residential staff from all the local authority social service departments in the area, or other similar agencies.

On a number of counts it would clearly be quite impracticable for all these people to meet together on any occasion in order to discuss the evolution of the service as a whole.

Where hierarchical organization exists it is appropriate that the senior person in the part of the hierarachy directly concerned with psychiatric services should speak for his or her subordinate staff. One may expect any manager to be able to take an appropriately broad view of integration and development, and it is quite in keeping that he or she should have authority to commit their own staff to action.[4] It is also possible that the senior manager from any hierarchy may require the support of a selected few of his or her immediate subordinates in any discussion or decision process, but so far as these people were concerned, such a discussion would in-

[4] Leaving as a separate issue any consultation which the senior manager might have with his or her own staff *en masse*, or through elected representatives, before undertaking discussions with people from other branches of the service.

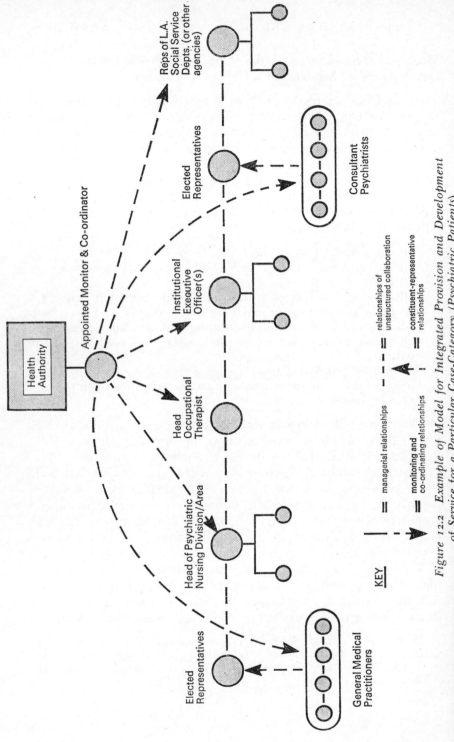

Figure 12.2 Example of Model for Integrated Provision and Development of Service for a Particular Case-Category (Psychiatric Patients)

KEY

—— = managerial relationships

– – – = monitoring and co-ordinating relationships

- - - = relationships of unstructured collaboration

⊢ = constituent-representative relationships

evitably have the underlying character of a 'command meeting'.[5]

Such a mechanism would usually apply therefore in nursing, in occupational therapy, and in social work. It would apply in relation to junior hospital medical staff working in psychiatry under the direction of a consultant psychiatrist. It would apply in relation to administrative staff.

It could not apply, however, to consultant medical staff as a whole, or to general medical practitioners, since their internal relationship is non-hierarchical. On the other hand, sheer weight of numbers would make the inclusion of all or a significant proportion of these people quite impossible, so that if their voice is to be heard in discussion it can only be through the mechanisms of elected representatives. As for the hierarchy, the one will speak for the many; but the difference between the manager and the elected representative is crucial, since the elected representative, unlike the manager, will not necessarily be in a position to commit his or her colleagues, or to make decisions which are binding on them.

However, it seems that by one or other of these means a manageable group of people might be assembled to discuss the provision and development of services, to allow mutual communication of problems, and to begin to form policies which were testable with their constituent members. Many such groups have indeed been formed in the past under titles such as 'maternity liaison committees' and 'geriatric liaison committees'.

But how can the health authority be sure that such work gets done, and gets done as well as might be? True, they can brief the heads of various hierarchies who are accountable to them, but they cannot brief any elected representatives, or review their work. Elected representatives take their brief from their constituents, and (in their representative role) are accountable only to these constituents, not to the health authority. And then another problem arises. Even if policies are agreed by such a group, and approved in turn by the health authority and the local social service authority, who is to translate the agreed policies into action?

The answer to both these problems may be for the health authority to appoint one person to act as their agent in this situation, with (at least) monitoring and co-ordinating authority. Such a person would certainly carry out the secretarial work in relation

[5] See Newman and Rowbottom (1968), Chapter 5.

to any meetings, and might or might not act in addition as chairman. He or she would be accountable to the authority for initiating discussions, where necessary; for providing data and carrying out any research necessary to illuminate discussion; for taking whatever action was necessary to implement any policies which were in fact agreed, and for monitoring the performance of individuals in relation to such agreed policies.

The desirable qualification or experience to carry such a role would be a debatable point. It is possible that one of the elected medical representatives might also double as an appointed co-ordinator, but some degree of role-conflict might well arise in this situation. In any case, there would be an awkward lack of continuity were one of the medical groups to elect as a new representative a person whom the local health authority considered unsuitable to act as their appointed agent.[6]

None of the individuals or groups concerned would of course be accountable to the co-ordinator. This would equally apply to any local authority social workers concerned in discussions. However, to the extent that policies on provision of services had been agreed by both the health authority and the local social service authority, there seems no reason why the co-ordinator could not continue to act *across* the organizational boundary in relation to any matters within the scope of joint policy where the prime problem lay with the health authority – say, for example, the procedures for 'handing-over' psychiatric patients on discharge from hospital to the care of local authority social service departments.

Models of Organization for the Integrated Provision and Development of the Services of Occupational Groups

The third field in which it is possible to consider integrative mechanisms is in relation to the work of occupational or professional groups – doctors, nurses, paramedical workers of various kinds, architects, engineers, accountants, and so on. Evidently, it is not part of the operational work of any health authority to create opportunities for employment and career progression for any

[6] The parallel between this discussion and that of 'Cogwheel' organization will be obvious – see Chapter 5. In a very real sense the discussion here is about the notion of an extended 'division' which includes representatives of *all* groups who have to do with a particular category of patient.

category of staff. On the other hand there must be consideration of the needs (and abilities) of particular occupational groups if effective operational work is to continue in the long run. More specifically, there must be systematic action in relation to each particular occupational group[7] in the following matters:

- basic professional training, and recruitment to the profession (if this is relevant);
- recruitment and induction to the health service;
- continued professional training thereafter;
- the issue of technical instructions and policies, or the dissemination of research findings relevant to professional practice;
- monitoring of professional standards achieved;
- negotiation of any special conditions of service (e.g. shift systems in nursing);
- career-planning within the health service.

(here 'profession' stands for 'profession or occupation').

Over and above organizing for these occupationally related activities, it may be desirable to organize for the production of certain operational or supportive services on an occupational basis. This suggests two main alternative organizational models, which are shown in Figure 12.3(a) and 12.3(b).[8]

In Figure 12.3(a) the basic workers in a particular occupational group are included within a hierarchical organization in each particular institution (hospital or health centre). The local head of the occupational hierarchy, if there is one, is immediately subordinate

[7] How far does the concept of occupational group spread? In common sociological usage it would include not only the 'major' professions – law, medicine, the church, but also the 'semi-professions' (vide Etzioni, 1969) – nursing, teaching, social work, etc., and indeed any working group that shared some common identity – clerical work, cleaning and portering. In terms of the present discussion, the concept virtually defines itself as any group in relation to which it is deemed necessary to make special organizational provision to deal with the needs listed here. Cleaners, for example, are a group for which the hospital has found it necessary to set-up special organizational arrangements for occupational integration. On the other hand 'clerical staff' as such, are not, or at least not as yet.

[8] The analysis here is similar to that used in relation to the multi-level organization of various existing hospital departments, in Chapter 8. Only the two main alternatives of local monitoring and co-ordination (outposting) or functional monitoring and co-ordination are examined in detail but, as in Chapter 8, the two other possibilities of attachment or secondment might also be explored.

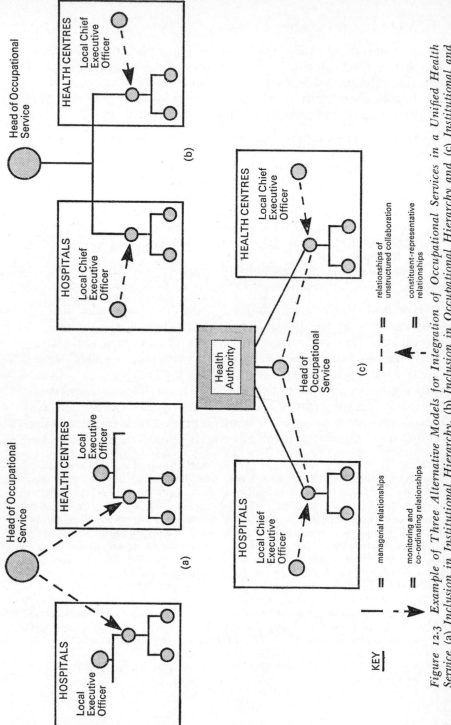

Figure 12.3 *Example of Three Alternative Models for Integration of Occupational Services in a Unified Health Service* (a) *Inclusion in Institutional Hierarchy,* (b) *Inclusion in Occupational Hierarchy and* (c) *Institutional and Occupational Monitoring and Co-ordination*

to some designated chief executive officer for the particular institution, whose own professional background might not necessarily be the same.

Assuming that it was considered necessary to establish integration across a number of institutions in relation to the sorts of occupational issues listed above, then a 'head of occupational services' post would be established at the next organizational level. Local occupational heads would not be subordinate to this person, but subject to his or her (functional) monitoring and co-ordinating authority in the way described in Chapter 4. Fieldwork in existing hospital organizations has shown for example that the relationship between many R.H.B. chief officers and their H.M.C. counterparts conforms to this pattern, as suggested in Chapter 10.

Alternatively (Figure 12.3(b)) the local staff in a given occupational group might be subordinate to the head of the occupational service, and thus part of one large hierarchy for the authority as a whole, with outposting arrangements to particular institutional sites. Here, the head of occupational service would be accountable not only for occupational monitoring and co-ordinating, but for the full management of the group, and for the services produced, whether they were technically operational activities or supporting services.

The local executive officer in this situation would no longer be in superior-subordinate relationship to the local occupational staff, but would play an (institutional) monitoring and co-ordinating role in the way described in Chapter 4. This is a common mode for the organization of occupational groups, and frequently arises, for example, in nursing, in engineering and building, and in physiotherapy and occupational therapy.

There is, however, a third organizational alternative, where the head of a local occupational hierarchy is subordinate neither to the local chief executive nor to the head of the service (Figure 12.3(c)). This applies currently in the case of consultant medical staff employed by R.H.B.s, whose work is co-ordinated on a local or institutional basis by an executive officer of the particular institution concerned, and regionally by the regional head of the service, the Senior Administrative Medical Officer.

Models of Organization for the Integrated Provision and Development of Services within Institutions (Hospitals and Health Centres)

The fourth field in which there is an obvious need for integrated mechanisms is the work as a whole of hospitals or health centres.

Whatever integrative mechanisms exist for co-ordinating the treatment of individual patients in a unified health service, there will continue to be the need to see, for example, that the multitudinous services on a hospital site come together in a co-ordinated way and are developed in a co-ordinated way: that various out-patients' services are arranged at compatible times; that new medical services are not launched without the backing of adequate nursing and paramedical services; that beds are not left regularly empty in one ward, whilst another ward is full to overflowing; and a thousand and one other things. In short, the individual hospital itself, and no doubt the health centre on a smaller scale, is a complex social entity in its own right, whose parts demand co-ordination and whose staff, being in a continuous position to react to each others' attitudes, work loads, conditions of service and morale, require 'managing' as one group.

For the sake of illustration, the various possibilities for integration within a single hospital will be examined, and then the extra complexities where the organization of hospitals in groups is envisaged.

The question of the best means of achieving integrated hospital management has a long and battle-scarred history.[9] On the whole it would be fair to generalize the trends of the nineteenth and early twentieth century as showing public hospitals coming increasingly under the control in each case of one medical director or superintendent; whilst the control in the voluntary hospital tended to be split amongst the doctors, the secretary (administrator) and the matron. In effect, the voluntary system prevailed; and (with possible exceptions in the case of certain small hospitals and psychiatric hospitals) the general pattern of hospital administration following the introduction of the National Health Service was the so-called 'tripartite' one. (The full significance of this in practice

[9] See for example Abel-Smith's authoritative account of the evolution of hospitals through the nineteenth century and up to the advent of the National Health Service (Abel-Smith, 1964).

has been explored in various aspects, in Part II).

The reason for the prevalence of the more complex administrative pattern of the voluntary hospital over the simpler public hospital pattern is probably to do with the gradual increase in the range of advanced medical and associated specialists working in most hospitals. Where the range of medical specialties employed in any hospital is small and the development of each is comparatively rudimentary, it is possible to find one doctor whose knowledge can readily comprehend each of them, and who then readily stands in a full-managerial relationship to the other medical practitioners and paramedical ancillaries, not to say to nursing and administrative staff. Other doctors then become his assistants. The modern specialist consultant does not fit easily into this pattern. He may have his own assistants but cannot be subordinated to a higher medical 'manager' without losing the essence of his role (see Chapter 5). Where then, a large number of consultants are associated with one large general hospital, as in the typical modern pattern, there is no possible one person to act as the manager of all medical services, and therefore, to some extent, no obvious figure to act as managerial director of all other services.

Many of the schemes for bringing about integrated management of the hospital under one 'managing director' or 'general manager'[10] fail to the extent that they ignore this particular social characteristic. If one accepts this characteristic as 'given' then the two polar extremes of possible organizational models are as illustrated in Figure 12.4.

Leaving aside the consultants for the moment, the 'unified management' model assumes that it would be possible to organize all hospital staff other than doctors in one hierarchy under some suitably-qualified chief executive officer. That is, the heads of the

[10] See for example the proposals worked out in some detail for hospital management under one 'general manager' contained in the King Edward's Hospital Fund Report (1967): *The Shape of Hospital Management in 1980?* True, the authors emphasize the need to maintain clinical freedom in individual case treatment (para. 54) but the implication elsewhere is that the general manager would carry full-managerial authority in relation to four 'Service Directors' and (presumably) in the last resort to all staff of the hospital, medical and other. Farquharson-Lang (1966) too, argue for one 'chief executive' for each category of board (para. 212), though little is said of what this signifies in terms of exact authority or role-relationship to doctors or any others.

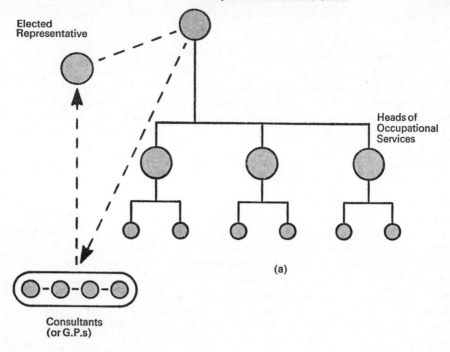

Hospital Chief Executive Officer

Elected
Representative

Heads of
Occupational
Services

(a)

Consultants
(or G.P.s)

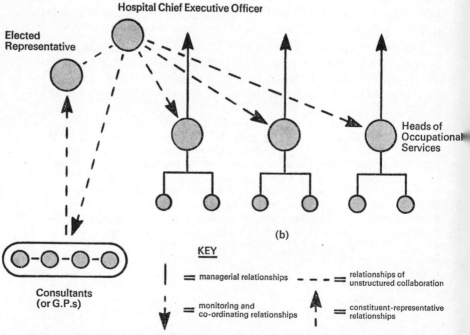

Hospital Chief Executive Officer

Elected
Representative

Heads of
Occupational
Services

(b)

Consultants
(or G.P.s)

KEY

= managerial relationships

= monitoring and
co-ordinating relationships

= relationships of
unstructured collaboration

= constituent-representative
relationships

*Figure 12.4 Example of Alternative Models for Integration of the Service
of a Single-Tier Hospital System (e.g. a District General Hospital) (a) Unified
Management and (b) Multi-Management*

various main occupational groups, other than any who were directly subordinate to doctors, would be directly subordinate to the hospital chief executive officer. This might include the Hospital Treasurer, the head nurse, the Hospital Engineer, the Building Supervisor, and so on. (The heads of certain smaller occupational groups – porters, and laundry staff, for example, would not necessarily be directly subordinate to the chief executive, but might be placed at one level further down in the hierarchy.) The hospital chief executive officer might also have immediately subordinate to him (but not shown in Figure 12.4) certain deputies and assistants.

The question of the appropriate qualifications for such a chief executive post would be a very significant matter. It would be one thing to declare that the occupant was managerially accountable for all the activities performed in the hospital other than those managerially controlled by doctors. The real question (as discussed in the previous chapter) would be whether a person could be found, or trained, who could reasonably be expected, not to have the ability himself to be able to perform all the variety of activities proposed by his subordinates, but certainly to be able to appreciate any problems which they might raise, however technical, in whatever depth was necessary, and to be able to make an adequate assessment of their work, technical aspects and all.

In any event it is likely that he would be supported by specialist staff from a higher organizational level, who would in this instance carry a functional monitoring and co-ordinating role in relation to the various heads of occupational services in the way described in the previous section.

As far as the medical staff of the hospital were concerned, three things need to be said. First, that each consultant would in general himself be the head of at least a small hierarchy of junior medical staff. In addition, in certain specialties (for example pathology) the consultant's subordinates might also include a relatively large number of paramedical staff (see Chapter 6). Secondly, the hospital chief executive officer, though clearly not in managerial relationship to consultant staff would be the obvious person to carry out a local monitoring and co-ordinating role in relation to the activities of consultant staff within that particular hospital, on behalf of the employing authority. The same remarks would apply to situations where general practitioners rather than consultants treated their own patients in hospital. Thirdly, it is likely that the consultants (or general practitioners) as a whole, would wish to express their views on the running of the hospital as a whole, through the mechanism of some committee and representative structure. This structure would in principle be different from any divisional structure as it would be related not to a 'division' of medicine, but to a particular site. It would be in fact the true hospital medical staff committee.[11]

It follows that the role of elected medical representative (or representatives) for the hospital should be most clearly differentiated from the monitoring and co-ordinating role. It is likely that the local medical representative and the local hospital co-ordinator would work most closely together, but in the last resort one would be accountable to his colleagues for expressing the consensus of their opinion on any issue, whilst the other would be accountable to the employing authority for ensuring within the limits of his authority that medical activities are kept within certain limits, that they are co-ordinated as well as possible, and that they are developed in as systematic a way as possible.[12]

[11] Division is used here as defined in the 'Cogwheel' Report. Any 'divisional' structure of medical staff would in fact be more closely related to the question of integration of what we are calling 'category of cases' services; and the analysis previously outlined would have direct relevance.

[12] This distinction perhaps throws new light on the old arguments about the need for medical superintendents or medical administrators in hospital. The *first* need is to decide whether one is talking about a representative role, or a monitoring and co-ordinating one. Assuming the latter, much of the heat disappears from the argument when the distinction between 'monitoring and co-ordinating' and full management is made. There then remain two real questions:

(a) should the monitoring and co-ordinating role in relation to medical work be filled by a practising consultant, or by a lay administrator?

(b) what is the full range of duties to be comprehended in monitoring and co-ordinating in relation to medical work?

On the first question, the Bradbeer Report (1954) opted for a consultant, and were applauded in their view by Guillebaud (1956). Scottish practice had always favoured a 'medical superintendent', who probably borrowed some additional authority from the Group Secretary, in comparison with the English and Welsh situation – see Acton Society Trust (1955): *Hospitals and the State, No. 3 Hospital Management Committees*, particularly Appendix VIII *Actual Duties of a Scottish Group Medical Superintendent*.

The second question has been discussed in Chapter 5. Naturally, the questions of exactly what are the duties, and what are desirable qualifications to carry them out, are clearly linked.

At the other extreme (Figure 12.4(b)) the hospital chief executive's role would be a monitoring and a co-ordinating one, rather than a managerial one, not only in relation to medical staff but in relation to the heads of all the various occupational groups within the hospital – the head nurse, the Treasurer, the engineer and so on. He might command his own direct assistants, but otherwise he would have no immediate subordinates. In essence (whatever his title) he would then be chief site co-ordinator, but there is no reason to assume that his work as such would be any less demanding than it was as a full manager in relation to a larger group of staff. In either situation the same *kinds* of work would be envisaged; programming and attempting to implement new projects; the collection, interpretation, and discussion with hospital staff, of operational data; handling of complaints; public relations work with the local community; acting as secretary to local committees, and so forth. What would be mainly different would be the degree of authority to prescribe the work of others, to apply sanctions as a result of assessment, and to initiate transfer or dismissal; and in consequence the degree of accountability for the work of others.

In between these two polar extremes would of course be a variety of intermediate possibilities in which differing numbers of groups of hospital staff were subordinate to, rather than co-ordinated by, the local chief executive.

Extension to a Two-Tier Hospital System

The variety of possible models for the integrated organization of a one-tier hospital (or health-centre) system can readily be extended to cover situations where hospitals (or health centres) are arranged in some group-structure (see Figure 12.5). For example, even with the growth of district general hospitals, large numbers of small hospitals are likely to continue in existence for many years to come, and it may well be convenient to incorporate these for administrative purposes in groups around a central district general hospital.

The two main alternatives again are those where the group or hospital chief executives carry a full-managerial role in relation to all staff other than consultants and their subordinates, and those where the group or hospital chief executives carry a monitoring and co-ordinating role in relation to these staff, though again the

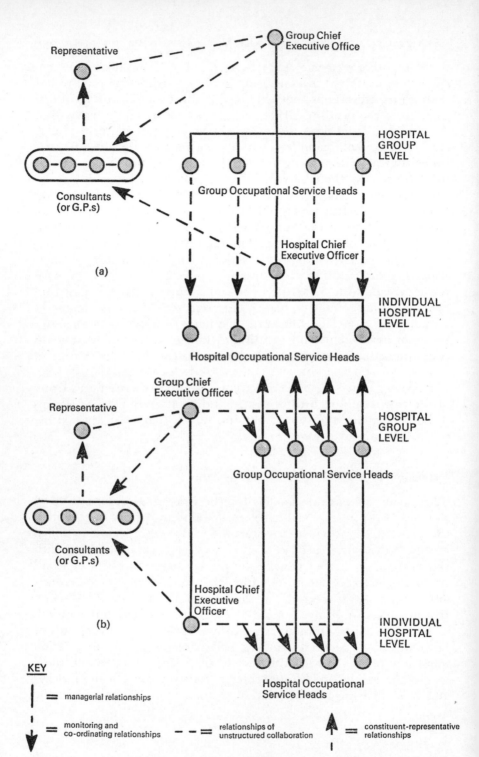

Representative

Group Chief
Executive Office

HOSPITAL
GROUP
LEVEL

Consultants
(or G.P.s)

Group Occupational Service Heads

Hospital Chief
Executive Officer

(a)

INDIVIDUAL
HOSPITAL
LEVEL

Hospital Occupational Service Heads

Group Chief
Executive Officer

Representative

HOSPITAL
GROUP
LEVEL

Group Occupational Service Heads

Consultants
(or G.P.s)

Hospital Chief
Executive
Officer

(b)

INDIVIDUAL
HOSPITAL
LEVEL

Hospital Occupational
Service Heads

KEY

= managerial relationships

= monitoring and
co-ordinating relationships

= relationships of
unstructured collaboration

= constituent-representative
relationships

*Figure 12.5 Examples of Alternative Models for Integration of the Service
of a Two-Tier Hospital System* (a) *Unified Management and*
(b) *Multi-Management*

further alternative possibilities of attachment or secondment could also be considered.

In the first case (Figure 12.5(a)) the unified-management situation, the group chief executive would have as his immediate subordinates all the group heads of occupational services, as well as the chief executive officers at particular hospitals. (The possibilities for staff-officer structure are considered later.) At hospital level the local heads of occupational services would probably then for the main – by the same organizational logic – be subordinate to the hospital chief executive officer, though in particular cases they might be directly subordinate to their corresponding group-heads (this latter situation is not shown in Figure 12.5(a)). Even where the first situation prevailed, however, the group occupational heads would undoubtedly still interact directly with their hospital counterparts, but the relationship would be functional co-ordination rather than superior-subordinate.

In relation to medical staff and their associated departments, the group chief executive officer would play an overall monitoring and co-ordinating role on behalf of the employing authority, and would need to work closely with the elected representative or representatives of all the medical staff who worked in the group. At the same time, to the extent that monitoring and co-ordinating of medical work was necessary at individual hospital level, as distinct from group level, the hospital chief executive officer would be the obvious person to assume the necessary role. It might well be that medical staff would need and want to set up a committee structure and representative system at individual hospital level, as well as at group level, in some cases.

In the second case (Figure 12.5(b)) the 'multi-management' case, the group chief executive would have only the following as direct subordinates:

(a) hospital chief executive officers;
(b) a small central secretariat of direct assistants.

Heads of occupational services at hospital level would be directly accountable to their group counterpart, and the latter either to more senior counterparts still at the next organizational level where such existed, or to the employing authority itself. Group chief executive officers and hospital chief executive officers would then play for the most part a monitoring and co-ordinating role.

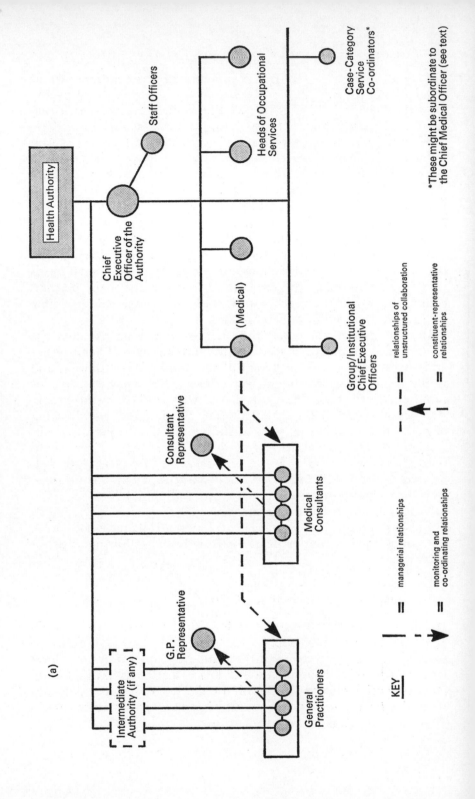

(a)

Health Authority

Chief Executive Officer of the Authority

Staff Officers

Heads of Occupational Services

(Medical)

Case-Category Service Co-ordinators*

Group/Institutional Chief Executive Officers

*These might be subordinate to the Chief Medical Officer (see text)

Intermediate Authority (if any)

G.P. Representative

Consultant Representative

Medical Consultants

General Practitioners

KEY

managerial relationships

monitoring and co-ordinating relationships

relationships of unstructured collaboration

constituent-representative relationships

(b)

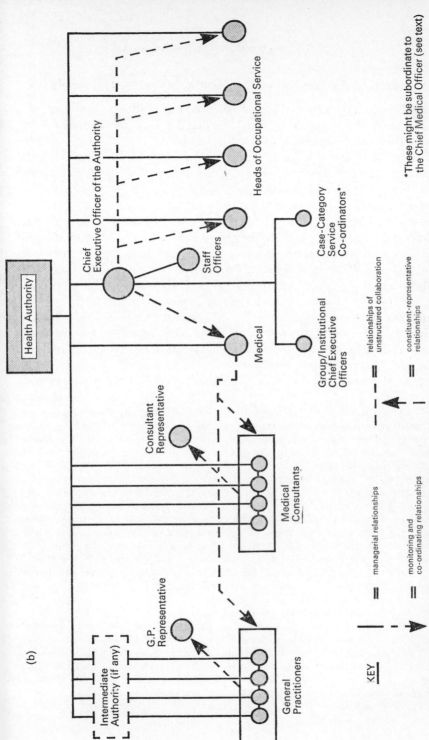

Health Authority

Chief Executive Officer of the Authority

Heads of Occupational Service

Staff Officers

Medical

Consultant Representative

Medical Consultants

Intermediate Authority (if any)

G.P. Representative

General Practitioners

Case-Category Service Co-ordinators*

Group/Institutional Chief Executive Officers

*These might be subordinate to the Chief Medical Officer (see text)

KEY

managerial relationships

monitoring and co-ordinating relationships

relationships of unstructured collaboration

constituent-representative relationships

Figure 12.6 Examples of Alternative Models for Integration of the Services of a Health Authority (a) Unified Management and (b) Multi-Management

Integration of the Services of the Health Authority as a whole

Finally we may consider mechanisms for the integration and development of the services of any health authority as a whole. Let us consider for example possible models for organization of a single district Area Health Authority in a new unified service. Again there are the two polar extremes of unified- and multi-management (see Figure 12.6) with a number of intermediates.

In all cases, it is assumed that general practitioners and consultants would form separate committees through which their views, ideas and reactions could be expressed. (The question of the existence of any intermediate authority for the employment of general practitioners is ignored for the purposes of this discussion.) The means of expression would be both through the publication of the minutes of the committee and also through the personal medium of elected representatives. Communication would be both with the committee of the health authority itself, and (more regularly and informally) with the chief executive officer of the authority, and the chief medical officer.[13]

It is also assumed that this chief medical officer would carry out

[13] The existence of elected medical representatives might allow any variety of 'management groups' or 'executive committees' to be established, bringing together these representatives, the chief executive and other principal officers, and even selected members of the governing body, to form a group to deal with any problem of management of the authority as a whole, within policy established by the governing body.

United Oxford Hospitals with the help of the McKinsey management consultants are reported (Sleight, Spencer & Towler, 1970) as having successfully established such an executive committee in a Board of Governors situation. The executive committee consisted of four medical representatives (three who were chairmen of the three medical divisions which had also been formed, and one from the medical staff council) the Chairman of the Board of Governors, the chairman of the Finance Committee of the Board of Governors, the director of nursing, a board member responsible for nursing, and the chief administrator of the Group.

Although such bodies may be called 'committees' it should be borne in mind that they are not true committees in the sense defined in Chapter 4. Majorities cannot outvote minorities. Administrators cannot overrule doctors or vice versa. People carry their usual roles, and usual organizational relationships into such situations, and to this extent the existence of such groups should be understood as elaborating existing organization rather than as creating new basic organization, though this does not necessarily detract from their usefulness.

all the functions of head of occupational service described above in relation to recruitment, training, clinical-policy setting, and general monitoring of service-standards. He would not of course be in superior-subordinate relationship to practising medical staff employed by the authority (as distinct from any medically quali- fied assistants of his own), but would act in an overall monitoring and co-ordinating role on medical activities throughout the author- ity. This is in addition to whatever other duties he might have as a community physician in relation to epidemiological work, plan- ning of new health facilities, provision of preventive medicine and health education, and provision of health advice to local authori- ties.

In relation to the chief medical officer and other heads of occupa- tional services – the chief nursing officer, the chief architect, the chief engineer, etc., chief executive officer of the authority might stand as a full manager (Figure 12.6(a)) or as a monitor and co- ordinator (Figure 12.6(b)). Any executive officers with administra- tive duties in relation to particular institutions (health centres, hospitals) or groups of institutions, would be subordinate to him. Also, were any class of full-time 'patient-group' co-ordinators brought into being, in the way described earlier in this chapter, then it is possible that they also would be subordinate to him. If these were doctors however – community physicians for example – it is perhaps more likely that they would be subordinate to the chief medical officer.

Conclusion

The main object of this chapter has not been to prescribe or recom- mend any particular organizational form, but to show rather how the elements evolved in project-work allow the construction of a *variety* of explicit models to meet different social, geographical and technical situations. It is certainly likely that in the complex situation of any large health service, with many professions prac- tising on many distinct sites, no one simple mechanism of organiza- tion will bear the work of the many kinds of co-ordination to be achieved.

13   Some Open Issues

At any moment of time in continuing project-work of the kind that has been described here certain issues are seen with comparative clarity, they have been fully analysed and alternative solutions fully tested in discussion, if not in the field. Other issues are just emerging on the horizon. They are dimly seen and not well understood, though perhaps of great potential importance. This chapter will be devoted to reporting such issues as they now appear.

Broadly they fall into two categories. The first are concerned with what might loosely be called 'management-structure' or more precisely, with the structure of the *executive role-system* (see Chapter 4) established by a health authority in order to get its work done. The second category of issues might be described as those of control and participation. They are to do with the functions and composition of the governing body itself, its relation to the community and to any higher authorities. Such considerations naturally extend to questioning how the views of constituent professions and occupations as a whole may be represented in policy making, and also how the grievances of individual members of the service, or members of the public served, can be adequately voiced and adequately responded to.

The Organizational Division of Operational and Other Activities

One large, and still as yet clouded, issue as regards internal role-structure might be put thus: what general models (if any) can be established for the division of activities within the total executive role-system of any health authority? Is personnel work, for example, a universal, and universally separable, component of work in health organizations, as in all other authorities? Is 'secretarial' work something essentially on its own, and different from 'medical administration'? What is the work of a 'functional head' and how does it relate to these other kinds of work? And so on.

The division of activities into 'operational' and 'other' (or 'non-operational') forms perhaps a useful starting point. For large, physically-spread, and comprehensive, health services such as the new National Health Service some partial generalization is possible, drawing on the fact that they are all likely to be concerned with co-ordinating operational activities for many kinds of clients, on many sites, delivered by persons of many skills.[1] As far as this kind of categorization is concerned, various alternative models were posed in the previous chapter.

Another possible generalization of operational activities might be in terms of the various stages into which they fall in any cycle of evolution of an operational service:

(1) research into community needs, and the evaluation of the extent and adequacy of existing services;[2]
(2) the planning and development of new or modified services;[2]
(3) the actual delivery of developed services.

Following on this, a possible categorization of other or non-operational activities might be as follows:

(4) the provision and maintenance of personnel resources – recruitment, training, welfare, negotiations with unions, etc.;
(5) provision of material resources and supporting services of various kinds (logistics)
(6) managerial-type work (as carried out in managerial, staff, supervisory, co-ordinating, or monitoring, roles) – the specification of duties and tasks, allocation of resources, reviewing of results, etc, (see detailed list in Chapter 4);
(7) financial work – cashier duties, the keeping of accounts, the production of financial forecasts and budgets, the monitoring of actual expenditure, etc;

[1] This is somewhat reminiscent of the possible alternative modes of organization considered by 'classical' management writers such as Gulick and Urwick (1937) into division by purpose, process, clientele, place. The point was made in the previous chapter that in regard to the health services, organizational machinery of some kind is needed to co-ordinate operational activities in all these dimensions.

[2] There is currently much discussion as to whether these particular activities should properly or usefully be classified as 'operational' or 'non-operational'. Their direct concern with operational matters suggests one answer. Their feel of 'back-room' or 'headquarters' work suggests the other.

(8) the provision of 'pure' secretarial services – servicing of committees, preparation of agenda and papers, production of minutes, communicating committee decisions or requests, carrying out legal work;

(9) public relations work.

Further questions now arise. Do these particular divisions of work reflect a natural division of roles? Would operational research and development (items 1 and 2) be the natural prerogative of a chief medical officer? Would personnel-provision (item 5) naturally associate with organization-development and specification (one of the elements of item 6)? Or would organizational-development (and training) be appropriately split amongst heads of occupational groups, in relation to members of their own occupations? Is the regular association in public-services of 'pure' secretarial work (item 8) with many 'management-type' activities (item 6) an unquestionable one?[3] Where do 'management-service' type staff (operations researchers, work study staff, systems analysts, organization and methods officers etc.) fit into the picture?

These and similar questions await further clarification. Before passing on, however, the views on this topic expressed in the First Green Paper (Ministry of Health, 1968) are probably worth reconsideration. There a five-fold general management division at Area Board (sic) headquarters was suggested, as follows.[4]

[3] As remarked before it is usual in commercial enterprises to have both a secretary and a chief executive – the managing director (Gower 1957, Ch. 1). In this situation the separation of 'pure' secretarial work and 'executive' work is readily observable.

[4] The military precedent was clearly influential. In the British Army for example, apart from the commander, the chiefs of technical troops and directors of administrative services (rather akin to the heads of occupational services described) the threefold division of staff-officers is: –

(a) staff-officers of the Adjutant-General's Branch of the staff (personnel work);

(b) staff-officers of the General-Staff Branch (intelligence – i.e. field research – operation and training); and

(c) staff-officers of the Quartermaster General's Branch of the Staff (supply). – (see Dale and Urwick, 1960)

The extent to which the military model is translatable to the health field is obviously an open question. An alternative conception of staff-officer roles as being essentially of three kinds – personnel, technical, or programming, was developed in the Glacier Project (Brown 1960). (See the more extended discussions of this latter conception in Chapter 4.)

'The organization of the Area Board's headquarters should also be such as would ensure the comprehensive planning and management of services. The desirable form of organization seems to be a functional one. There might be four or five major departments:

(1) Planning and operation of services: maintenance and development of unified services; planning of new capital projects; research and statistics; and liaison with the services of other authorities.
(2) Staff: personnel and staffing matters; establishments; training; recruitment; careers; and contracts for service – with special emphasis on securing the optimum use of staff throughout the service.
(3) Logistics: supply; construction and maintenance of building and engineering services and equipment; and transport.
(4) Finance: estimates; accounts; costing and cost/effectiveness analysis.
(5) Secretariat: including headquarters and senior establishment work; management services; and public relations. (Possibly in smaller Areas this could be combined with the Staff Department at (2) above.)'

Links with tentative categories established above will be obvious.

The Function of Governing Bodies in Public Health Services

Other issues loom, on broader questions of participation in, and control of, any health service as a whole. In any national health service, for instance, what are the specific functions for which it is necessary to establish statutory authorities with corporate governing bodies at various levels? Could these functions in principle not be carried out equally well through an executive-system of appointed officers?

It is easily said that governing bodies must be responsible for policy and officers for administration, but harder to produce any convincing and water-tight distinction between these two activities.[5] At the same time some real and important distinction no

[5] The Maud Report (1967), greatly concerned with relationships between officers and members of public authorities (in this case local authorities), having taken expert advice pronounced categorically that definition of the distinction between policy and administration was not only impossible but indeed undesirable (paras. 109, 143) The Farquharson-Lang Report (1966),

doubt exists, otherwise the choice of a system of local health authorities as opposed to a single monolithic organization under the Secretary of State in the National Health Service would hardly have arisen as a real one (as it obviously is, whatever the merits or demerits of the two alternatives).

Our own preliminary analysis of this mattter is as follows. Any distinction between policy and administration is certainly not one of who makes the decisions. The supposition that officers merely 'carry out' – in a totally prescribed way – the decision made by the authority itself is so obviously naïve that detailed refutation is unnecessary. All work involves decision-making, though it is clearly the case that decisions of the governing body set a framework for more detailed decision-making by officers. Nor on the other hand is the work of the governing body distinguishable from the work of the executive by supposing that the former make all decisions on matters of value, whereas the latter decide only matters of fact or method. The fact is that *all* decisions, at whatever organizational level, and however far-reaching or trivial, necessarily involve some element of value-judgment.[6]

Our hypothesis for the moment is that the distinction is indeed real, and that it turns on the authority to make value-decisions of a particular kind – in the health field, decisions about the kinds and priorities of health services required by the community. It is, arguably, the function of the governing body to crystallize the otherwise unexpressed norms of the community[7] in regard to matters like:

– the relative priorities to be given to various existing medical services (say, maternity as against mental subnormality);
– the priorities to be given to the development of new services (e.g. renal dialysis);

---

concerned again with the same relationship but now in the hospital field, leaned heavily on the distinction in general terms (paras. 51 onward) without however attempting the job of precise definition.

[6] As convincingly demonstrated by H. A. Simon in *Administrative Behaviour* (1957), one of the pioneer works in decision-theory.

[7] This is not to suggest that systematic data on needs, and indeed opinions, could not and should not be collected wherever practicable, quite apart from data on the adequacy of existing services. What is suggested here, however, is that it is the peculiar function of the governing body to make the final evaluation – the final value-judgments – where the facts and opinions leave off and the action begins.

- the tolerability of various lengths of waiting times for various services;
- appropriate standards of food and accommodation for inpatients;
- appropriate patterns of patient-visiting times; and so on.

In all such matters the governing bodies would require information and advice from officers, both lay and medical, but it is suggested the final decisions would be theirs and theirs alone.

It follows of course, that the governing body must also make the final decisions on allocation of resources, once more with due guidance on costed alternatives from officers. Again, it would be the duty of the governing body not only to set standards in these matters, but to see in practice that these standards were adhered to. Gathering these ideas together, than, a skeleton descripion of the specific functions of a governing body in the public services might read as follows:

(1) Defining in general terms the kind, standards and priorities of operational services required.
(2) Determining the general allocation of resources.
(3) Appointing and assessing chief officers.
(4) Reviewing standards actually achieved and money actually spent, attempting to ensure adequate performance in practice.

Governing bodies make the ultimate decisions on services required and priorities – the political decisions – but they do not themselves have to execute the operational tasks which follow from these decisions. They need a high degree of sensitivity to the many hues and varieties of community opinion. They do not need to have a high facility to create plans, to pursue and elaborate alternatives, to conduct long negotiations or to provide continuous supervision of current work. The issues facing them, when properly defined, are relatively simple in terms of decision-making processes (though not necessarily in terms of political implications). The appropriate social form is many-personed, where each contributes some special knowledge of, or sensitivity to, the multitudinous needs and problems of the community and of the service.[8]

[8] This suggests that the National Health Service Reorganization Consultation Document (Department of Health and Social Security 1971) in advocating that management ability should be the main criteria for selection of members of the new authorities (para. 14) might have failed to recognize an important distinction in kinds of personal qualities needed. 'Administrative man' and 'political man' may well be quite different animals.

On the other hand, the executive system (see Chapter 4) which supports the governing body does perhaps need a high capacity to carry out just these detailed interacting and continuous activities mentioned above. It does not need the same wide and sensitive receptivity to broad and sometimes ill-defined social needs if the governing body is doing its job. But it must above all be able to act in a controlled and co-ordinated way. It cries out for the individual chief executive or chief co-ordinator, and tends (where other social features allow) to the hierarchical form.[9]

With this in mind, the role of chairman could perhaps be more clearly distinguished from the role of any one chief executive, or the executive roles of a number of separate chief officers. The role of chairman characteristically involves, of course, the direction and control of meetings of the governing body itself, but it also involves acting between meetings as the voice and eyes of the committee. Where rapid guidance was needed in *political* decisions (in the sense of decisions which reflect community values) as opposed to executive decisions, then it would be recognized as the chairman's job to give such guidance – subject to the later review of the governing body in full.

Appointed and Elected Governing Bodies

Such discussion inevitably leads on to a further issue – what is the organizational significance of the governing bodies in public services whose members are appointed by higher authorities (for example existing H.M.C.s or future Area Health Authorities) in contrast to those whose members are elected by a local community (for example, existing county councils)?[10] Could anything be said

[9] Again, 'hierarchy' is used here in the precise and limited sense defined in Chapter 4, and is not intended to carry connotation of either an authoritarian or for that matter a permissive social atmosphere or managerial style.

[10] Compromises are possible, with mixtures of appointed and elected members or with combinations of elected members from quite different bodies of constituents, for example local electorates and professional groups. Examples of such intermediate bodies are provided by the existing Executive Councils who administer general practitioner services – see Chapter 2, also the composite Area Health Authorities proposed in the Second Green Paper – Department of Health and Social Security, 1970b. All such composite bodies suffer a fundamental constitutional weakness. Governing bodies are strongest when they are able to act as true committees, i.e. on a majority

about the kind of public service that lends itself to one organizational form rather than another? Again, the issues are largely unexplored in project-work at this stage. However, it may be useful to note, at least for the moment, three basic alternative ways in which a national service may be run, with either elected or appointed authorities (see Figure 13.1).

Firstly, services to be provided may be conceived nationally and administered in one large national executive system, with appropriate outposting of staff to local offices (Figure 13.1(a)). Currently, national employment services are run in this way. All political decisions are made by central government. All executive action is carried out by the Civil Service, and it is left to the judgment of individual officers of the service to adjust local practice and policies to local needs and circumstances as they think fit. Where hierarchical organization of this kind arises, there is a maximum concentration of accountability for the operation of the service as a whole at the topmost level.

Secondly, the services to be made available may be defined in broad terms by central government, but actually provided by elected local authorities (Figure 13.1(b)). Currently, social services, for example, are organized in this way. This system provides for maximum sensitivity to local needs and views, under the final direction of a national governing body but, as has been well observed,[11] leaves a tenuous authority-link between the central and local levels, and in consequence weakens the concentration of accountability.

Here, the influence of central government is largely limited to:

(a) its authority to legislate;
(b) its authority, stemming from legislation, to direct or approve decisions in certain key areas, for example in senior appointments in some services, or generally on capital expenditure;
(c) its authority to persuade or advise through publication of circulars, or the personal intervention of professional groups such

---

vote, rather than as unstructured coalitions, which need unanimous agreement. As was discussed in Chapter 4, the committee-form supposes an underlying unanimity of interest amongst members which can only be a reality if all are appointed by one person or authority, or elected by one integral group of constituents.

[11] See Griffiths (1966).

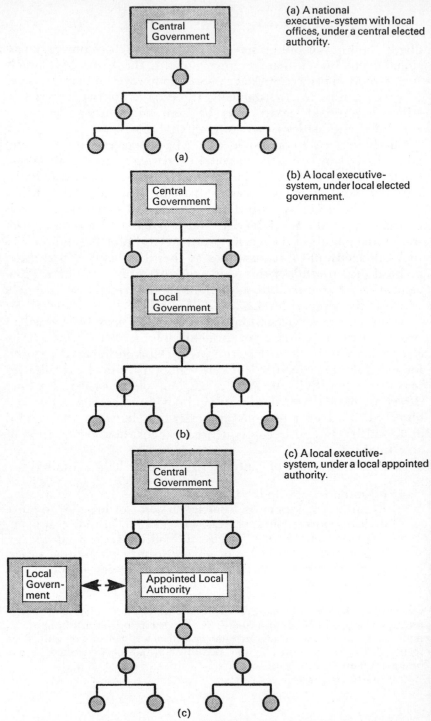

(a) A national executive-system with local offices, under a central elected authority.

(a)

(b) A local executive-system, under local elected government.

(b)

(c) A local executive-system, under a local appointed authority.

(c)

Central Government

Central Government

Local Government

Central Government

Local Government

Appointed Local Authority

Figure 13.1   Three Alternative Structures for National Public Services

as the Social Work Service, or the H.M. Inspectorate (in education);[12]
(d) its authority to allocate or withdraw financial support.

In the case of the National Health Service though, it appears
that the third form above (Figure 13.1(c)) is the preferred one.
Within this frame of analysis this form can be viewed as an attempt
to combine some of the enhanced sensitivity of the second form to
variations in local needs and standards with some of the central
concentration of authority and accountability of the first.

However, given the existence of subordinate authorities with a
separate legal identity and constitution, defined in statute, there
can never be a relationship exactly managerial in quality between
successive tiers. Higher bodies may have authority to direct, and
perhaps even to make arrangements for alternative provision of
services in 'default' circumstances, but there can never be the
straightforward ebb and flow of work between superior and subordinate that naturally and regularly occurs in any managerial
relationship.

Subordinate authorities will have their own statutorily-defined
functions, and if higher authorities are not satisfied with the way
they are carrying them out they will rely on persuasion, pressure,
or in the extreme case formal direction or even reconstitution of
the membership of the authority. What they will not readily be
able to do in such circumstances will be to involve themselves
directly and undramatically in the management of any service at
fault, to the extent in effect of bringing some of the burden of the
work of provision back on to their own shoulders. In effect, they
will not easily be able to say (as can an individual manager to his
individual subordinate) 'here, let me show you how to do this' or
even 'here, you had better leave that to me'.

The Representation of Staff and Consumer Interests

If health authorities *are* appointed by the Secretary of State
(directly or indirectly) one thing is clear: they cannot then properly be described as *representatives*, either of the communities in

[12] Owen (1971) provides an interesting analysis of relations between central
government and local authority, and in particular has perceptive comments
on the important function of a central inspectorate-cum-advisory service.

which they provide services or (naturally) of the staff they employ.
Thus a further series of as yet unexplored issues lies in this area.
How are health authorities, if at all, to be sure that the views of the
local community are represented in their deliberations? How are
they, again if at all, to be sure that the views of their own employees
too are represented?

As a first shy at the earlier question, the real problem is to find
a realistic method of election of community representatives, assuming again that such are required. Of course, if spontaneous pressure-
groups emerge, either national (like those concerned with
particular needs, for example, mental health) or local (as in the
case of any spontaneous neighbourhood councils which may
emerge) then representatives will readily exist, but they will only
be representative of those who happen to be members of their
associations. Leaving aside any possibility of the direct election of
'health representatives', one is inevitably driven back to the fact
that the place where genuine elected representatives of local committees are most readily to be found is in existing local authorities
themselves. Is it too much to envisage an arrangement whereby
health authorities systematically test the acceptability of their plans
and actual performance against community opinion through the
medium of some joint council, in which members of health authorities meet members of the local authorities themselves?[13]

As far as staff-participation is concerned, it has already been
pointed out that whilst officers can *present* the opinions of their
subordinates, as well as they are able to judge them, they can never
realistically *represent* their subordinates. Only freely-elected representatives can do that. Again the main problem is to find some
workable system of representation. It is only too easy for some
management-created system to be set up, in which duly-elected
actors go obediently through their laid-down roles, steering away
from forbidden topics (such as pay); but this means little unless
there is some real flesh and blood movement from below, creating
its own representatives and expressing its own immediately-felt
problems. That such systems are possible in principle is amply
evidenced by the vigorous and universal existence of medical-
representative machinery in hospitals, as well as by those few

[13] In the precise language of the research, such bodies would not be true
committees – neither side could 'outvote' the other – but a *coalition* or
collegiate (Chapter 4).

hospitals that have successful Joint Consultative Councils.[14] So far our own project-work in this area has been slight.

Review and Grievance Systems

Finally, various systems for independent review, or for dealing with grievances of staff or patients are still an uncharted area in the research.

In fact, one is probably dealing with two organizational phenomena here – systems for the general review of standards of work on the one hand, and systems for handling grievances on the other.

It is of course part of the function of any responsible body or person to review the work of their subordinates, individual or corporate. Any ward sister checks the work of her nurses from time to time without any special ado, just as any governing body asks from time to time for progress reports from its officers. The place where special review machinery seems to be needed on occasion is at higher levels, between successive tiers of statutory authorities. Between the Secretary of State and subsidiary hospital authorities lies at present, for example, the Hospital Advisory Service, which in spite of its name is clearly designed to play a monitoring or review type role of in addition to any advisory role.[15]

Even at this level, however, the existence of such special machinery presumably does not relieve the Secretary of State or his officials from making from time to time their own personal and direct reviews of the work of the service for whose administration they are accountable.

In the same way, of course, it might no doubt be argued that dealing with grievances from patients or staff is also part and parcel of any managerial or directing role. Certainly this was the view of members of the H.M.C. who participated in the project-discussion described in Chapter 10. Nevertheless, there is always some role-conflict for members of executive-systems or governing bodies who deal with complaints – hence the agitation for independent

[14] The uneven history of joint consultation in the hospital service is examined by Miles and Smith (1969) in a survey of 200 hospitals. They report that most of the consciously-created Joint Consultative Councils which were initiated in 1950 have since foundered.

[15] See Department of Health and Social Security Circular HM (70) 17. Obvious similarities exist between this body and, for example, the HM Inspectorate in education or the Social Work Service in social services.

'ombudsmen'. Inevitably in such situations the member concerned is in some degree playing both defendant and judge.

Even without independent machinery, however, there is probably room for the evolution of some more formal procedures for dealing with complaints within the present framework; with due divorce from normal executive processes on the one hand, and from the too-blunt instrument of full representative machinery on the other.[16] Again, this area of organization still remains for exploration.

Conclusion

It is as well to conclude by emphasizing again the speculative nature of the material discussed here, unlike the material described in Part II, which has grown from actual field-projects and been subjected to considerable further test and discussion in steering committees and conferences. The aim of this chapter was to mark out as clearly as possible some of the areas which now appear ripe for project-work, or in which project-work has as yet only barely started. Increasingly now the scope extends beyond the detailed working of the executive system of hospitals to the broader fields of participation and control – the general relationships of the hospital to its social environment, the community, the professions, and government.

[16] One has in mind here for example, the explicit separation of appeals processes from both executive processes and representative or 'legislative' processes, adopted by the Glacier Metal Company, as described by Brown (1960).

14 Retrospect and Prospect

As was remarked at the beginning, this book is essentially a progress report on a continuing project.

At the time of writing, various hospital groups involved in the work are at the stage of embarking on experimental changes in, or redefinitions of, organization; and all these are viewed as 'pilot' schemes in the sense that the outcomes will be scrutinized with interest by higher hospital authorities for evidence of their more general applicability. On the other hand, the sweep of the project-work now begins to broaden and change direction, as the object shifts from hospitals to a total health service.

Two things this project-work is not – as it is hoped the presentation given here has by now made clear. Firstly, it is neither simply a systematic survey nor a series of case-studies of the present organizational state of hospitals or any other part of the service, although it is in some respects descriptive in nature. But neither is it simply a prescription for how hospitals or the health service might be better organized, although the project is certainly concerned with change and improvement.

Essentially the project-work is a continuing collaboration of members of the service with analyst-researchers and the job of the latter is to help the former clarify their own organizational values and the organizational means through which these values may be most effectively realized.

At the very deepest level the most important outcome is the shared insight of officers and analysts into the possibilities offered by the collaboration. In practical terms the research so far can be seen to have produced:

(1) A number of definitions of basic concepts with which to apprehend the stuff of organization itself – role, duty, task, authority, accountability, sanction etc. (as set out in Chapter 3).

(2) At the next level, a number of 'building-blocks' of requisite organization defined in terms of these basic concepts, each formed, tested and agreed in various different field-project situations – 'managerial', 'monitoring and co-ordinating', 'service-giving', 'representative', 'treatment-prescribing' roles, and so on – in larger sub-assemblies, 'executive hierarchies', 'governing committees', 'coalitions' and representative structures of various kinds (as set out in detail in Chapter 4).

(3) At the next level again, a number of agreed statements of how these building blocks are currently best assembled to meet various situations of existing hospital organization, in nursing, medical and paramedical organization etc., and for hospitals as a whole (as discussed in Chapters 5-10).

(4) Finally, illustration of how these blocks may be reassembled in various ways to integrate and co-ordinate various kinds of health service provisions (Chapter 12) given a variety of social, technical and geographical requirements.

It is in the hope that this accumulated material will already be of significant use to those who at various levels will be deciding the shape of the British National Health Service (as well as other health services elsewhere) that we have broken from our field-work to present it here, unfinished though it is.

Appendix A. Glossary

The origin and fuller significance of the various concepts listed below are explored in Chapters 3 and 4. Definitions are reproduced here for easier reference *in alphabetical order*.

Accountability

Accountability is an attribute of a *role*. It means that the occupant of the role is likely to be subject to positive or negative sanctions according to assessments of his work-performance in the role.

Appeals or Grievance Procedures

An appeals or grievance procedure is any which allows an individual (user or employee) to have reviewed his complaint against specific actions of a public service on grounds of departure from policy, irregularity, impropriety or inequity. It is to be contrasted with group action through *representatives* by which consensus opinions can be brought to bear in a policy-making situation.

Assessment

1. Informal assessments of people's work performance can be and are made by any number of fellow workers, but assessments made by *superiors* (or any others) with authority to sanction as well, have an obvious and special significance. Thus it is one thing to express an informal opinion about the performance of a fellow worker, but quite another to have the authority to record that opinion in such a way as to affect his prospects of promotion.

2. Assessments of work performance may be of two kinds:

    2.1 Assessments of *quality* or *adequacy* of the work of the performer, that is, of the quality or adequacy of his exercise of discretion.

    2.2 Assessments of the *regularity* of the work of the performer, that is, whether or not it conforms to policy, regulations and law. *Assumed* (see Manifest).

Attachment (see also Secondment and Outposting)

1. When a specialist function exists at different levels of an organization a junior specialist (BS) may be required to serve under the command of a non-specialist (B), while at the same time remaining the subordinate of a specialist superior (AS). The junior specialist thus has two superiors who are together accountable for his work to their common superior (A). This situation is described as *attachment*.

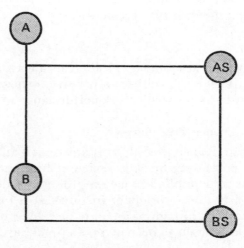

2. The specialist or functional superior AS is accountable:

    (a) for helping to select BS;
    (b) for the technical induction and training of BS;
    (c) for giving BS suitable technical prescriptions for his ongoing work;

3. AS has authority to give prescriptions on method to BS.

4. B is accountable for the substance of the work of BS and has authority to specify actual tasks and their priorities.

5. AS and B jointly assess BS.

6. AS and B each has authority to initiate the transfer of B. (Note: this definition is that officially established for the moment, in project-work. It is not quite in line with the analysis of attach-

ment presented in Chapter 4, and may need some further amendment in consequence.)

Authority

1. Authority is an attribute of a role. It is the right to act at discretion, as sanctioned by those who have *power* in the situation.
2. Authority may be to expend resources (cash, materials or human) at discretion. It may be to prescribe the work of others at discretion in some respect. Or it may be the right to apply sanctions to others at discretion, in some respect.

Coalition (or Collegiate)

1. A coalition is a co-operating group unstructured by mutual (organizational) authority, and in the absence of any external role with arbitrating authority.
2. Action on significant issues can only proceed with the agreement of all.

Collateral Relationships

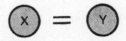

1. A collateral relationship is one where the work of two people ultimately subject to the authority of a common superior interacts in such a way that mutual accommodation is needed in certain decisions, and where neither has authority over the other.
2. Where collateral colleagues fail to reach agreement, ultimate resolution can only be found at the *cross-over point* represented by that common superior.

Committee

1. A (true) committee is a face-to-face co-operating group where it it agreed that action in disputed cases can be taken by majority decision.
2. This presupposes some strong basic consensus of interest amongst members, and usually means that they have been elected or appointed by the same group or body.

Co-ordinating Role

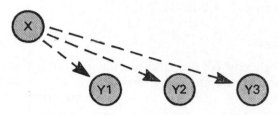

1. A co-ordinating role arises where it is felt necessary to establish one person, with the function of co-ordinating the work of a number of others in certain respects, and where a managerial, supervisory, or staff, relationship is inappropriate. The activity to be co-ordinated might for example be:

- the production of a report, estimate, plan or policy proposal;
- the implementation of an approved scheme or project;
- the overcoming of some unforeseen problem affecting normal work.

2. In all cases the co-ordinator can only work within the framework of some specific *task* whose definition is agreeable to all concerned.

3. Specifically, X in a co-ordinating role is accountable in relation to the task concerned for:

(a) negotiating co-ordinated work programmes;
(b) arranging the allocation of existing resources or seeking additional resources where necessary;
(c) monitoring (q.v.) actual progress;
(d) helping to overcome problems encountered by Y_1, Y_2 etc;
(e) reporting on progress to those who established the co-ordinating role.

4. In carrying out these activities the co-ordinator X has authority to make firm proposals for action, to arrange meetings, to obtain first-hand knowledge of progress, etc., and to decide what shall be done in situations of uncertainty, but he has no authority in case of sustained disagreements to issue overriding instructions. Y_1, Y_2, etc., have always the right of direct access to the higher authorities who are setting or sanctioning the tasks to be co-ordinated.

5. It is not part of the co-ordinator's role to make formal assessments of the general quality of the performance of those he co-ordinates.

6. There may be situations in which a co-ordinating role is played in part by a small group, e.g. a committee, rather than by an individual.

Cross-over Point

1. A cross-over point is the lowest role in an *executive hierarchy* where a common *superior* can resolve disagreements between colleagues in *collateral* or *service* relationships.

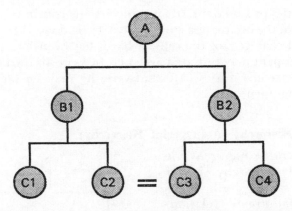

2. In the diagram shown, A is the cross-over point for any unresolved disagreements between C1 and C3.

Deputizing and Acting Management

1. In the absence of any *superior* from his normal phase of work, certain decisions may need to be made by one of his subordinates. Which decisions must be made, and which may be left for referral to the superior on his return will be determined to a great extent by the expected duration of absence of the superior.
2. One of the subordinates will need to be assigned this *deputizing* function whether or not the work 'deputy' figures in his role title.
3. Where the deputy in the absence of his superior takes on so much of his superior's role in relation to the other subordinates, as to be perceived as carrying accountability for their work, and as carrying authority to assess them and if necessary, to apply sanctions to them, *deputizing* changes to *acting management*. (This implication is that the deputy has the personal capacity to carry the full weight of his superiors's role, with the further implication that he

is unlikely to be satisfied with a diminished role on the return of his superior.)

4. It has not proved possible to assign any other significance to the word 'deputy' than that described above; that is, it has not proved possible to identify any function for a deputy as such, which survives the return of his superior.

Duties (or Functions)

1. The duties or functions, of any role are the continuing expectation made of the occupant as to the work to be done. They describe the general character of the role: what it has been set up to do.

2. The occupant may initiate particular *tasks* at his own discretion in response to his duties. Alternatively, he may be set tasks, by specific assignment.

Executive Hierarchy (Managerial Hierarchy)

1. An executive hierarchy, or managerial hierarchy is an *executive system* built upon *superior-subordinate* relationships. It therefore always has the feature of having one role at the top where the occupant is accountable for the work of all those under him.

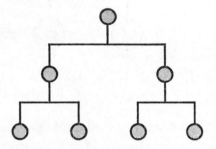

Executive System

1. An executive system is the system of roles in an organization which have the function of carrying out the work implicit in the objects of the organization.

Extant – see Manifest

Functional Monitoring and Co-ordination

(No agreed formal denition as yet exists for this relationship. See discussion in Chapter 4.)

Manifest, Assumed, Extant, and Requisite, Situations

1. The MANIFEST situation – the situation as it appears in charts, policy statement and the like.
2. The ASSUMED situation – the situation as each individual assumes it to be, before systematic analysis.
3. The EXTANT situation – the situation which actually exists, as it is gradually revealed by systematic discussion and exploration.
4. The REQUISITE situation – the situation which appears to meet most closely the various given needs and realities of the situation (for example, the work that is required to be done, the economic, environmental, and psychological, facts of the situation) as revealed by systematic analysis.

Monitoring Role

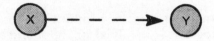

1. A monitoring role X arises where it is felt necessary to ensure that the activities of Y conform to adequate standards in some particular respect, and where a managerial, supervisory or staff relationship is impossible or needs supplementing. The field of performance being monitored might for example be:

- adherence to the letter of contract of employment (attendance, hours of work for example);
- adherence to the substance of contract of employment (quantity or quality of work produced);
- adherence to regulations;
- safety;
- financial propriety;
- level of expenditure;
- technical standard of work;
- progress on specific project.

2. Two broad categories of monitoring will be:

(a) monitoring in respect of adherence to limiting conditions (minimal standards, regulations etc.);
(b) monitoring in respect of standards achieved within limiting conditions.

Any given monitoring role may be concerned with the first only, or with both.

3. Specifically, X in a monitoring role is accountable for:

   (a) ensuring that he is adequately informed of the effects of Y's performance in the field concerned;
   (b) negotiating improvements with Y where necessary, or failing satisfaction, with Y's superiors;
   (c) reporting to the higher authorities to whom he is accountable sustained or significant departures in the field concerned;
   (d) recommending definitions of standards or changes to standards where required.

4. The monitor X has authority:

   (a) to obtain first-hand knowledge of Y's activities and problems concerning adherence to the limiting requirements;
   (b) to persuade Y to modify his performance, but not to instruct him.

5. The monitoring role is often combined with an advisory role where special expertise is involved in the monitoring function.

6. It is not part of the role of the monitor to make formal assessments of the general quality of Y's performance – this is the prerogative of the managerial role, if such exists.

7. It is possible that roles exist which carry out some but not all of full-monitoring functions. A *scanning* role, for example, might be established in order to provide information about actual performance in the field concerned, without having also the function of evaluating deviations or of negotiating improvements.

8. There may be situations in which a monitoring role is played in full or part by a small group of people, e.g. a committee, rather than by an individual.

Operational and Non-Operational Activity

1. Operational activity is that which arises directly out of the given objects of the organization – activity in providing the services that the organization is in existence to provide.

2. Non-operational activity is all the activity needed to support this – provision of resources, provision of accounts, maintenance of records, etc.

Outposting

1. A subordinate may be posted to work in a division of the organization which is functionally or geographically separate from that of his superior. When the original superior remains fully accountable for the work of the subordinate the situation is called *outposting*.

2. In this situation it is requisite that the original superior retain all the components of superior authority over the subordinate and that the superior accountable for the division in which he is outposted have none, other than that of requesting removal of the subordinate if his behaviour adversely affects the situation under the command of the second superior.

(Note: this definition probably requires amendment to give more explicit recognition of the monitoring and co-ordinating role of the local site superior – see Chapter 4.)

Policy (see also **Task**)

1. Policies are continuing prescriptions which limit or guide work. Some limit discretion without directly implying the creation of separate *tasks* (example 1: 'employ only qualified staff for this post'). Others (*duties*) imply that *tasks* have to be initiated to put them into effect (example 2: 'Better provision should be made for mentally subnormal patients').

2. Policies can be very general (example 2) above or very specific (example 1 above). Whether general or specific they are distinguishable from *tasks* in that, lacking specific reference to time limits, they do not in themselves define specific pieces of work to be done.

Power

1. Power is an attribute of an individual or a group, and indicates the ability to act or cause action at discretion (in contrast to authority, which expresses a sanctioned right to act at discretion).

2. Power rests therefore on personal qualities – personality, knowledge, expertise and so on – and on the possession of appropriate resources.

3. Effective organization thus rests both on structural factors

(appropriate authority) and personal factors (having competent people in roles with adequate resources).

Ranks and Grades

1. Discussion of hierarchy must distinguish between the structure of executive ranks in superior-subordinate relationships to ensure effective control of performance, and the structure of grades to ensure appropriate payment and possibilities for the progression of individuals. More grades than ranks may be necessary. The following diagram illustrates this difference. Once this distinction is made it becomes possible to see that a higher grade does not necessarily confer authority over a lower one.

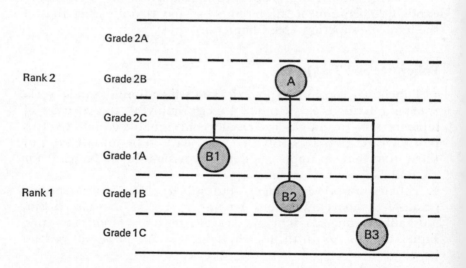

Representative Roles

1. Where any group wish to express the consensus of their views, or to negotiate with any other body, they may choose to do so through the medium of an elected representative.

2. The representative will be accountable to the group for what he says and does, but will need some degree of discretion in presenting views or negotiating. If he is judged inadequate by them the group must be able to replace him.

3. It follows that no true representative of a group can be appointed by a body or authority external to the group.

4. The term representative may also be used of an individual appointed by an organized body to voice their opinions and interests in dealings with other groups or bodies.

Representative System

A representative system is one in which a number of *representatives* of different groups or bodies (including particular groups of employed staff) interact in order to communicate the views of those they represent, to reach common policies, or to negotiate.

Responsibility

1. Responsibility may be thought of as a personal attribute – having a sense of responsibility – in contrast to *accountability*, which is an attribute of an organizational role.

2. Just as effective organization requires people with the personal capacity (power) to use the authority in their roles, so it requires people with an adequate sense of responsibility to accord with their accountability in role.

Role

1. *Role* may be briefly described as a set of expectations of behaviour in a given social situation.

2. Organizational roles can usefully be explored and defined in terms of:

   (a) the *duties* or *functions* which fall to the occupant;
   (b) the *discretion* or *authority* available in carrying out these and the various limits to it which exist;
   (c) (sometimes) the particular *tasks* which structure activity in the role;
   (d) the *accountability* of the occupant for his performance.

Secondment

1. A superior may transfer one of his subordinates to the command of another officer for an agreed period of time or for the duration

of a project. When the superior to whom the subordinate has been transferred is accountable for all of the subordinate's work the situation is called *secondment*.

(The definition of the term 'secondment' in the Salmon Report differs from that given here.)

2. The superior to whom the subordinate has been transferred will carry authority:

(a) to prescribe his work;
(b) to report his assessment of his work to the original superior;
(c) to initiate his re-transfer should his work prove unacceptable.

3. The original superior will retain authority to record formal assessments and to initiate permanent transfer in view of his on-going relationship with the subordinate.

Sanction

1. To sanction some action or performance is to prevent or approve it, to censure or reward it.
2. All sanctioning rests on *power*, but within an organization one can also talk of the *authority* (i.e. right) to employ sanctions resting with a particular role.

Service Relationship

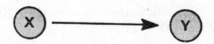

A service relationship is one where:

1. X may request, at his discretion, services from Y within certain limits on the kinds of services to be made available.
2. Y is accountable for providing such services within the limits of his own resources, and policies on the kinds of services available.
3. There is a common superior at the *cross-over point* who can receive any unresolved questions of quality or priority of service, and can set common policies within which both service-seekers and service-givers must operate.

Staff Relationship

1. A superior (A) may need assistance in co-ordinating the activities of his subordinates (B1, B2). Such assistance may be needed on personnel and organizational matters, on the programming of activities and services, on the techniques to be employed, and perhaps financial matters. The superior may establish in any of these dimensions a subordinate role whose occupant has authority to

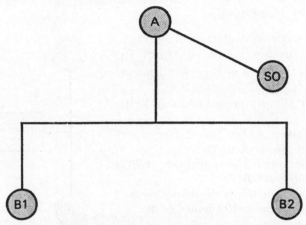

interpret the superior's policy to his other subordinates and to give instructions within that policy. Such a role is called a *staff officer*. The relationship between the staff officer (SO) and other subordinates (B1, B2) is called a *staff relationship*.

2. If B1 does not agree with the staff officer's interpretation he cannot disregard it, but must take the matter up with A. A remains accountable for the work of B1 and B2 and the staff officer.

Superior-subordinate Relationship

1. A superior-subordinate relationship is one where A is accountable for ensuring that certain work is carried out and has a subordinate B to assist him in this work.

2. In this situation it is requisite that A should have authority to:

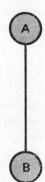

(a) prescribe B's work and assign tasks to him;
(b) veto the appointment of B to the role;
(c) apply sanctions to B (for example: record assessments of performance in such a way as to affect B's future career);
(d) initiate the transfer of B from the particular role he carries, where he judges his performance not to reach an adequate standard.

Supervisory Relationship

1. A supervisory relationship arises where a manager A needs help in managing the work of his subordinates B1, B2, etc., in all its aspects.
2. Specifically, the supervisor will help A:

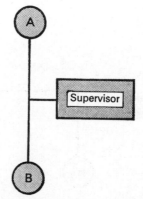

(a) to induct B into his duties;
(b) to assign work to B;
(c) to deal with the immediate work-problems of B;
(d) to monitor the performance of B;
(e) to assess the performance of B.

3. The supervisor has authority to prescribe the work of B but will not have the right of veto on the appointment of B, the right to apply sanctions to B, or to initiate his transfer or dismissal.

Task (see also Policy)

1. A task is a piece of work with a specific objective which is to be met within some definite time scale.
2. Within an *executive system* tasks may arise:

(a) at the discretion of the performer, in response to some (continuing) duty;
(b) by specific assignment.

3. Even where they are initiated at the discretion of the performer, individual tasks within an executive system must conform in scope and time-scale to the limits allowed by the executive system.

Treatment-prescribing Relationship

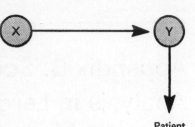

1. A treatment-prescribing relationship arises where X (a doctor, say) has authority to prescribe the treatments that Y must give to a patient.
2. X must deal with queries on treatment posed by Y and *monitor* the treatments actually being given.
3. X is not in a superior-subordinate relationship to Y. Y may use discretion in carrying out the prescriptions and may delegate specific treatment tasks to his own subordinates. Y is accountable to his own superior for observing treatment-prescriptions and for the discretion exercised in applying them.

Appendix B. Social Analysis in Large-Scale Organizational Change

The project described is perhaps remarkable for the sheer size of organizational study and systematic change with which it has become concerned. The work in the North West Metropolitan Hospital Board Region, which forms a large proportion of the total activity of the project, is now concerned with the systematic development of organization throughout the whole Region, which employs about 30,000 people in twenty-three groups of hospitals.

A general indication of the method of work employed, and the machinery of Local, Regional and National Steering Committees which guides the work was given in Chapter 1. In this Appendix, certain aspects of the method will be elaborated, and the first outlines of a total strategy for forwarding large-scale organizational change of this kind, based on 'social analysis' will be described, as it now begins to appear.

The method will be related to other methods of social research and change, and an attempt will be made to answer the two crucial questions 'does it really achieve change?' and 'is it really scientific?'[1]

Main Characteristics of the Project Method

The method used in the project is taken from that employed by

---

[1] Of course, no one outcome can at the same time be both practical (i.e. change-producing) and scientific (i.e. knowledge-creating) in itself, but the question is whether this particular process gives rise to outcomes of both kinds.

Jaques in the Glacier Project. In a definitive paper Jaques (1965) summarizes what he calls the 'social analytic'[2] approach as follows:

'In essence, then, social analysis requires an individual or individuals in an organization, with a problem concerning the working of the organization, who seek the help of an analyst in determining the nature of the problem. The analyst is independent in the sense that he is not personally embroiled in the organization and its problems; he is from outside. He offers analytical help; he does not urge a particular course of action. The individuals in the organization also remain independent: they decide what they are going to do, and do it. It is not for the social-analyst to arrogate to himself either the authority or the accountability of those with whom he is working.'

Three aspects of this description warrant emphasis: firstly the collaborative relationship of the researcher (or analyst) and the organization member (or client); secondly the essentially analytic role of the former; and thirdly the concern with *organizational problems* rather than with personal ones. Let us examine each in turn.

Collaboration

The collaborative character of the association between researcher and client gives the researcher the inestimable boon of access in depth to the processes and problems or organization, but it also brings certain necessary (and sometimes, demanding) conditions.

Firstly, the privileged position of the analyst implies *confidentiality*; not just the condition that the analyst should not publish the specific material of discussion to the outside world, but that he should not divulge without permission material to members of the organization other than the particular client or particular group of clients with whom he is working at any one moment. All material is confidential to the individual client or group of clients up to the time when they specifically agree to release it. After this

[2] The term 'organization analysis' as used by Newman and Rowbottom (1968) refers to study of the same kind of subject material as that studied by Jaques and Brown in the Glacier Project (particularly in its later stages) but is concerned essentially with a particular mode of *thinking* about organization rather than with the *methods of collaboration and analysis* by which organizational knowledge in general may be extended and change produced.

point, the released material (but only this material) can be discussed with the wider group for whom it has been released. (Etymo-
logically, one remembers that 'confidentiality' and 'confidence'
spring from the same roots.)

Secondly, collaboration must by definition imply the unforced
agreement of the subject at all times of the continuing process,
his uncoerced and voluntary co-operation. It is only indeed the
presence of genuine collaboration that allows the subject at all to
be thought of as a 'client'. Now ensuring that co-operation is truly
voluntary can obviously be a tricky matter in an organizational
situation. Members of hospitals, like members of all organizations,
are liable to coercion of two kinds in this situation, whether the
coercion is overt or hidden. Firstly, there are pressures from
superiors. Where one's boss says 'would you like to undertake discussion with this researcher?' the question can never be as neutral
as it sounds. Secondly, there are social pressures from peers, particularly in meeting-situations. Who is going to be the odd man
out when all else agree to join the study?

Whilst these pressures are recognized in the project-work as an
inescapable fact of organizational life, at the same time every effort
is made to minimize their effects by emphasis on formal and sometimes seemingly elaborate procedures for establishing agreement.
For example, an attempt is always made at the start of a project to
establish some degree of agreement by the institution as a whole
for the commencement of work. Where bodies of a representative
kind already exist – staff committees, governing bodies, consultative committees, representative systems, or whatever – the analyst
will always gladly make use of them to give an opportunity to test
the general level of agreement throughout the institution (say, a
hospital) for social-analysis to be undertaken. Where such general
representative bodies do not exist, special 'project steering committees' have to be created, with as broad a representation as is
practicable, to carry out just this function.

At a second stage, much use is made of general explanatory and
exploratory discussion with large groups of staff – groups of doctors,
groups of midwives, selected groups of departmental heads, for
example – in order to create and test the general degree of agreement of particular groups with whom work has been suggested.
At a third stage, preliminary discussion is held with each individual, again to clarify the nature of the process to be undertaken

and to test the extent of his own personal agreement, before substantive project discussion is started. Finally, it is indicated to all individuals and to all groups who agree to participate that they still have the right to opt out should they wish, at any later stage. In fact, in the course of three or four years of project-work a number of individuals and a number of groups have chosen to discontinue project-work, sometimes making explicit their decision to stop, more often merely by letting discussions lapse.[3]

Analysis

The analytic character of the researcher/analyst's contribution is implicit in the basic collaborative association. Given the analyst's voluntary sharing of his client's concerns, but given also his lack of both executive authority, and accountability for executive results, it follows that either advice or analysis is all he could possibly offer. The exact difference between 'advice' and 'analysis' is perhaps difficult to establish, but assuming that the social-analyst does not make claims of any special knowledge or expertise in his clients affairs, and noting that he certainly cannot have a full knowledge and understanding of the total field-situation in which his clients' work, it seems preferable to think of his role as analytic, rather than advisory.

The analytic process with either individuals or groups can in fact be thought of as progressing through a number of definite stages, as suggested by Brown (1960) – consideration of the manifest, the assumed, the extant and the requisite situation. 'Manifest' here means the situation as formally and publicly displayed at the time of discussion, for example, in any existing directives or policy-statements. The 'assumed' is the first, unanalysed view of what the client actually believes, or what the group of clients believe, to be the case, which may or may not coincide with the manifest statement. Following analysis the client or group of clients may see, however, that the true existing organizational reality – the 'extant' situation – is different again. With existing reality exposed as far as is practical or possible the discussion can then naturally lead to

---

[3] Once again one must emphasize that since no question of representative sampling is involved here the number and kinds of people who elect to co-operate in project work, or who choose not to do so, has no statistical significance.

whether or not this is 'requisite' and if not, what changes would be necessary to make it so. (See also under 'Manifest' in Appendix A.)

This last concept is the most important. The 'requisite' is not a statement of the ideal or utopian, but a statement of what, *given certain constraints*, is considered to be the optimum. Releasing some of these constraints, the optimum may naturally change. For example, given a situation where staff skilled in the management of both engineering and building work were virtually unobtainable, the separate organization of building and engineering might be requisite. Were the constraints on the recruitment or training of jointly-qualified staff to relax, joint-organization might be more requisite.

Concepts of the manifest, the assumed, the extant and the requisite are all used in analysis, but as far as outcomes are concerned, it is statements of the *requisite* which are the target at all stages. Separate statements of 'manifest', 'assumed' or 'extant' situations are rarely if ever recorded, indeed without using role-concepts such as *co-ordinating* role or *managerial* role which themselves enshrine notions of requisiteness it is very difficult to make coherent statements of extant organization. (As suggested many times in the previous text the 'extant' organization needs to be created as much as described, given that one chooses to use these particular terms of description.) What frequently does happen, however, is that two levels of requisite statement are recorded: what would be requisite accepting certain existing constraints, and what would be requisite were these removed.

Kind of Problems Considered

The third characteristic of social analysis is its concern with organizational problems *per se*. (Note that Jaques uses the phrase 'problem(s) concerning the working of the organization' as part of the definitive statement quoted above.) What does or does not qualify as an organizational problem? As a matter of historical fact, as will have been evident from the previous text, the project-work so far in this hospital project has been concerned wholly with questions of organizational structure as defined in Chapter 3, i.e. with questions of individual role-functions and individual role-relationships and with questions of the functions (i.e. the operational activities) and role structure of the organization as a whole.

However, there is no reason in principle why organizational problems should be so narrowly construed.[4] The same approach of collaboration and analysis could readily be extended from organizational structure to organizational procedures – for example, planning and control procedures, recruitment procedures, buying procedures, job evaluation and grading procedures, staff appraisal and training procedures, and so on. It might conceivably be extended in certain cases to analysis of the basic operational technology employed by the organization – the methods of selling, product development, production, education, care, treatment or whatever.

One real limit is the point where a relationship which is simply analytic becomes inappropriate or ineffectual. This might be the case where the primary need was for the provision of hard advice rather than the provision of analysis, and where such advice was to be had, based on some established and accepted expertise, e.g. in the fields of law, medicine, engineering, computer technology, and so on. Alternatively, the real need might be for a data-collection exercise, or survey, the basic problem having already been analysed and diagnosed to the satisfaction of the sponsors (see later discussion).

Another limit is reached when the problem raised belongs really to the individual rather than to the organization – where the problem is really the individual's lack of ability, or his immaturity, or his psychological malfunctioning. Here, if there is work to be done, it is not work for the social analyst, but work for the educator, the doctor or the personal therapist. An interesting border-line case is work with the face-to-face groups where the analysis proceeds in terms of 'group-dynamics', i.e. work in the social-psychological area. To the extent that this work is really focused on the performance of a given group within a given organizational setting it could properly claim to be organizational, though the importance of

---

[4] Nor have they always been so in social analytic project work. The Glacier project-work included analysis of job-evaluation systems, and pricing procedures in a commercial company, for example (Jaques 1956, 1967: Brown and Jaques 1964). A current social analytic project in local authority social service departments being undertaken by the author and others (not yet fully reported) is analysing procedures for receiving, assessing and allocating cases requiring social work, to give another example.

consideration of the effect of given organizational role-relationships on group behaviour would always bear stressing. To the extent that the work was focused on improving the perception and perform-ance of the individual group-member it should really be classed as personal development, education, or therapy.[5]

Kinds of Activity Undertaken in Project Work

Experience within the hospital project has shown that a number of different kinds of collaborative activity become necessary as large-scale analysis and change proceed. So far activity of the following kinds have emerged:

(1) field-project discussions with individuals;
(2) field-project discussions with groups;
(3) research conferences;
(4) executive conferences;
(5) training conferences.

Discussions with individual organization members in designated field projects are the foundation of all project-work.[6] Such field-projects may be initiated by any member or organization. Desir-ably, suggested projects should be sanctioned by the institution as a whole, through the means, for example, of the local project steering committee where such exists. Assuming that the project is to involve a group of people rather than one individual, the next step, as described above, is to seek their joint agreement and finally

[5] The gradual shift from analysis focused on psycho-social characteristics to analysis focused on sociological concepts – the characteristics of institu-tionalized roles and procedures – is evident in the Glacier Project, for example, comparing 'Changing Culture of a Factory' with later works. The majority of 'planned-change' projects – see later section of text – on either side of the Atlantic have in fact tended to focus fairly strongly on small group behaviour, very often in groups formed outside the organizational context in 'T-group' or 'sensitivity training' sessions (Bradford, Gibb & Benne 1964). The comment that the attempt to change the individual's behaviour and perception is unlikely to be effective without reinforcing it by change in the organizational environment in which that individual is then to work, is an obvious one. (Katz and Kahn, 1965 – Chapter 13).

[6] Jaques (op cit) has elaborated the important reason for work with the individual as well as, and preliminary to, work with the group in project-work of this kind.

the agreement of each before individual discussions take place.

In the normal event, cleared material from these individual field-project discussions then flows for group-discussion by those immediately involved. Sometimes a series of cleared reports of individual discussions is circulated by the researcher to the group by way of preparation. Sometimes the researcher prepares and circulates a general report using cleared material from individual discussions as he thinks fit. Almost always, a series of discussions is required with the group before any definite conclusions can be reached. Finally, the best analysis that can be made of the situation together with any proposals on requisite organization reached by the group is then fed to other interested groups (or their representatives) or to the next level of responsible officers, or both, for further discussion and agreement. Eventually the resulting analysis and proposals are fed to the local steering committee for their test and agreement.

In one sense, changes start to take place from the first moments of the first discussion, for if the analysis is at all successful organization-members involved inevitably find themselves with some degree of change in their perception of their organizational situation and problems, and such changes in perception must necessarily alter their organizational behaviour thereafter in some degree or other, however small. At the same time the moment in any project when the proposals emerging from the project-work are approved by those in authority and can now be 'officially adopted' marks an obvious and important step in the change process. Indeed proposals which require changes in staff establishment or radical changes in duties may be quite impossible to implement in any degree before this point.

The third kind of collaborative activity that has evolved during the project is the *research conference*. Here, researchers meet groups selected to give a mixture of members from a variety of occupations and sites. The purpose of this event is twofold:

(a) to disseminate project-findings to a larger organizational group, and
(b) further to test and refine findings by exposure to group discussions and criticism.

(By 'project findings' is of course meant the cumulative analysis and formulation of requisite organization that exists at any time, at whatever stage of test and agreement it has already reached.) One hopes that each research conference will lead participants from the organization to a greater awareness of organizational realities, problems, and possible solutions, and give the researchers an increasingly accurate and tested understanding of these things too.

However, as project-work has proceeded, two rather more precisely-structured variants of the research conference have come to be felt necessary. The first is the *executive conference*. Here, a group of organization members are assembled with an explicit organizational problem in mind. The task may be to study their own organizational interactions. For example, groups of supplies officers have met with their area and regional chiefs to try and elucidate their requisite organization of supplies staff in their Region. Alternatively they may meet in order to clarify their ideas on organization policies with whose implementation they are all concerned. For example, groups of chief nursing officers have met with nursing staff from Regional Headquarters to elucidate possible regional policy on the general development of nursing structure along the lines of the Salmon Report (1966). As a direct result of executive conferences of this kind it is possible for researchers to summarize analysis and proposals so that further discussion and possible implementation can proceed as in field projects. Research conferences do not give rise to such direct project-work, though they stimulate better formulations of problems and possibilities in a number of other specific projects being undertaken at the same time.

The second variant of the research conference is the training conference, or more properly the *training course*. Here the aim is primarily to produce by the end of a course a group of people with an appreciably better understanding of organizational problems, possibilities, or policies, or with appreciably improved skills in some processes of organizational or social analysis. The supposition in genuine training is that the trainer has more to teach than he has to learn (though he is not in fact specifically precluded from learning!). In research conferences the contrary supposition is tolerable. A training conference then, assumes a relatively advanced stage of project-work where certain findings are held with considerable confidence following previous test in the conference or in the field.

Even if large-scale organizational change is to take place through the dissemination of explicit policy, large-scale training is un-doubtedly required as well to support the process. However, a research team, even a large one, could never hope to provide the full volume of training required to support the extent of change envisaged in this particular hospital project, which is no less than altering the perceptions and behaviour of the staff of a whole Region. One answer would seem to be for the research team to concentrate on training a group of trainers.

But it is likely that large-scale programmes of organizational change will require more even than general policy statement and widespread, general, training. It is likely that a whole cadre of specialists in organization analysis will be required within the organization itself, to cope with problems of detailed implementa-tion and development on each site. Where intensive project-work is being undertaken by the research team, such specialist skill is in a sense already provided, but again, such research support cannot possibly be made available at every site in the Region. The second training task, then, must be to train specialists in organization –

Table B1   The Successive Phases of Large-Scale Organizational Change

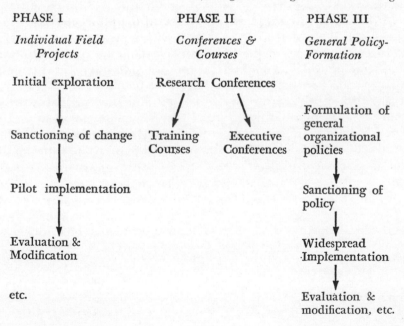

PHASE I	PHASE II	PHASE III
Individual Field Projects	*Conferences & Courses*	*General Policy-Formation*
Initial exploration	Research Conferences	
↓	↙ ↘	Formulation of general organizational policies
Sanctioning of change	Training Courses Executive Conferences	↓
↓		Sanctioning of policy
Pilot implementation		↓
↓		Widespread Implementation
Evaluation & Modification		↓
etc.		Evaluation & modification, etc.

administrators, personnel officers, management-services officers, and so on – to produce 'activists' within the organization itself.[7]

The sequence of these various activities as the project has proceeded has fallen into three broad and heavily overlapping phases, as illustrated in Table B1.

Individual field projects, involving discussions with individual clients and groups can be thought of as constituting the first phase. In the work described in this text some dozens of individual field-projects have now been undertaken, many of which have reached a point where proposals for change are about to be or have just been sanctioned for pilot implementation at the time of writing.[8]

Very early in the work, a second phase of activity commenced as the first of a series of research conferences was mounted, drawing on the preliminary material which had emerged from field projects (with due regard to anonymity). These conferences themselves acted as a form of testing. Following the approval in principle by the North West Metropolitan Board of some of the definitions of basic organizational concepts and of the first statements of organizational alternatives – the beginning of Phase III – it was possible to advance to more structured events – the executive conference and the training course.

At the time of writing it is expected that the policy-making body (the North West Metropolitan Board) will be in a position to make an increasing range of positive statements of policy on organization, which can be disseminated through the Region with the help of large-scale training, and particularly, as mentioned, the training of 'activists' in the form of organization and personnel specialists from each Hospital Group. Thus Phase II will continue and support Phase III. At the same time Phase I will continue too, as specific field projects are launched to explore new areas in depth, and as older field projects where pilot changes have already been implemented are evaluated and modified where necessary.

An intricate network of feedback now comes into existence to

[7] Unlike the people in the hospital project teams trained to carry out work in the Hospital Internal Communications Projects (Weiland 1971, Revans 1971), these would be people who were concerned with organizational development as a regular and continuing part of their work.

[8] The difficulty in the hospital service with its large and intricate national structure of getting agreement for explicit and in some cases radical changes to be tried was noted in Chapter 1.

put to good use the results of these various parts of the work. As individual field projects are launched, tested, and evaluated, their results inform and modify the proceedings in conferences and courses. Later conferences modify the ideas of earlier ones, and suggest in turn new ideas for trial in field projects. All these findings contribute to the formulation of general policy, and the results of the implementation of general policy also provide a source of feedback for the later modification of these same policies.

Comparison with Other Approaches

The social-analytic approach is easily confused with three other research approaches – the *survey*, the *case study*, and *participant observation*.[9] It has in fact, distinctive differences.

In a survey the definition of the problem to be explored and the relevant data to collect rests firmly with the researcher.[10] This gives him an ability to plan the collection of data, using sampling techniques of greater or lesser sophistication, in a way that simply is not open to the analyst in social-analysis. On the other hand two of the preconditions for successful survey-work are firstly, that the relevant data can be adequately defined and, secondly, that direct access to this data in its true form can be counted on. Given the typical problems tackled by social analysts neither of these conditions is likely to hold. Without the right conditions of access, and motivation for co-operation, any data immediately available would be trivial or worthless compared with that which results from the long and painful process of analysis and clarification – in the language of the method it would merely be manifest or at best, assumed data.

The case study is closer perhaps to social analysis than is the survey, but the orientation of the researcher is still that of any observer rather than that of a collaborative participant. The researcher is free to establish problems, pursue exploration and publish his own explanation and interpretations as he thinks fit,

[9] See for example the description of these methods by Goode & Hatte (1952).

[10] This would not be true of a commissioned survey, but even then the precise definition of problems to be explored and data collected will rest with those who commission or plan the survey, rather than with the respondents.

given some minimum degree of co-operation from those he studies in allowing him to observe and collect data in the first place. Again this is not a description of social analysis.

On the other hand participant observation in projects might be thought to go beyond the degree of participation established in social analysis. The participant observer by definition involves himself to some degree in the very activities he wishes to observe – whatever reserve he may inwardly and privately maintain, he becomes outwardly a member of the working group, with all the difficulties of maintaining due objectivity that this may bring. Of all breeds of social researcher he is prepared to pay the highest price for the valued gift of access.

In this respect the social-analyst stands as it were halfway between the case study observer and the participant observer. In the struggle to maintain both objectivity and access he offers participation of a kind – help and collaboration – but reserves the right to establish his own independent 'professional'[11] position.

The true genus to which social analysis belongs is not the survey, the case study, or participant observation, but what Lippit, Watson & Westley (1958) and later, Bennis, Benne & Chin (1969) have called the process of 'planned change'. (A direct social and historical link can be traced from this conception of 'planned change' to Kurt Lewin's earlier and related conception of 'action research'. Bennis[12] succinctly summarizes the essentials as follows. 'The process of planned change involves a *change agent* a *client system*, and the collaborative attempt to apply *valid knowledge* to the client's problems' (author's italics). Lippit et al. differentiate four main classes of 'client-system' – the individual personality, the face-to-face group, the organization and the community.[13] They thus draw attention to an essential similarity in the

---

[11] This outlook is institutionalized in the role of the practising professional – the doctor, lawyer, social worker – who must assume concern for the problem of his client, but at the same time must preserve his own independent and overriding value-system, the ethic or code of the profession.

[12] Op. cit. p. 65.

[13] Op. cit. pp. 5-9. They also suggest a number of typical stages in the process of planned change (p. 30).
1. Development of a need for change ('unfreezing').
2. Establishment of a change relationship.
3. Working towards change ('moving').
4. Generalization and stabilization of change ('freezing').

work of a diverse group of social caseworkers, psychiatrists, psycho-therapists, counsellors, group workers, community workers, management consultants and so on. However Bennis' definition also suggests that not just any helping relationship would qualify as planned change, but makes the application of valid knowledge a necessary element. Thus the change agent must be more than a man of action, he must be a professional who draws on a body of scientific knowledge. He, or some of his fellows, must also be concerned to develop this knowledge and its application, they must be in part researchers, scientists or technologists as well as prac-titioners.[14] (See notes on characteristics of profession – Chapter 5, Note 1).

It appears then that social analysis is an example of a process of planned change, distinguished from others only in its restriction of subject matter to problems of the functioning of organizations, as discussed above.

---

5. Achieving a terminal relationship.
(The terms in brackets refer to an earlier and broader scheme of Lewin's.)
In terms of the phases of project-work we have described above, stage 1 represents the initial approach of the researcher to various hospital groups; stage 2 the setting-up of steering committees and the preliminary approval of projects by institution, group, and individual; stage 3 represents the process of analysis; and stage 4 the process of pilot implementation, policy formation and training.
Bennis suggests that in practice, training, consultancy, and applied re-search, are the main tools of the change agent (op. cit. p. 70) – again the similarity to the project-work described above will be evident. He also suggests that the power of the change-agent to promote change stems not from coercion, tradition, or even expertise, but primarily from the values he exhibits. 'Most change agents do emit cues to a consistent value system. These values are based on Western civilization's notion of a scientific humanism; concern for our fellow men, experimentalism, openness and honesty, flexibility, co-operation and democracy' Op. cit. p. 74.
[14] There is a strong temptation, not to say tendency, for change agents to concentrate on action, and the science of action, at the expense of bringing any substantial science to the actual problems encountered. This criticism could be applied for instance to the Hospital Internal Communications Project (Weiland 1971, Revans 1971). Weiland comments (p. 34) that the essence of the project was to introduce survey-techniques to hospitals and adds (p. 357) that 'without a careful and clear diagnosis, including end-result, causal and changing variables, improvement of a problem situation is likely to be difficult, risky and probably temporary'.

Does Social Analysis Achieve Change?

Having identified social analysis as a 'planned-change' process we come to an obvious question: does it really achieve change in practice? Actually there are two related questions to be studied: does social analysis achieve change, and is the change in fact beneficial?

Before either of these questions can be answered, one important characteristic of social analysis must be stressed. The data with which it operates is not that of observed and recorded *behaviour* (verbal or physical) but that of observed and recorded *statements*. This is what collaboration means in this context: a series of discussions between researcher-analyst and one or more clients which result (typically) in recorded statements, be they statements of what is already manifest, of what is initially assumed, of what is later judged to be the extant reality, or what is later still judged to be requisite.

Given that clients *agree* statements, whether they in fact then act in keeping with these agreed statements at that time or subsequently, is another matter, and one which is in a sense outside the competence of the analyst to consider. If the client says he finds an analysis satisfactory and states that he agrees with its outcome, then the analyst is bound to assume that the client means what he says. He cannot possibly undertake an independent *check* of his client's behaviour without destroying the whole basis of the collaborative relationship.[15]

As far as the analyst-researcher is concerned, then, the prime information available to him of his effectiveness in changing his client's situation is his client's personal response, and in the last resort, the continuing interest of the client and his willingness to devote time and money to a continuing dialogue. In practice the important signals for the analyst of positive progress, however partial, are the moments when the client appears to commit himself with conviction to some new formulation or reformulation posed by the analyst. The signal of success is the moment agreement is reached.

[15] Though this does not *seem* to rule out the possibility in principle of a check by some third party in the form of observations of the changed behaviour of the client, or his improved performance: see discussion below on this point.

But what is the situation if the client is fooling himself? If the analyst's own intuition does not tell him (as it often does of course, particularly if a formulation does not quite ring true though the client is eager to agree) it is difficult for more to be said or done by either. And even assuming the existence of a third party in the role of observer, any further evidence of progress would turn on whether the observer's 'objective' reports were more 'real' than the stated feelings of progress of the involved client.

However to leave the argument simply at this is too cavalier. There must, in principle at least, be some possibility of the production of definite evidence of change or improvement, and to deny the possibility even in principle, is in effect to deny completely the place of measurement in human endeavour.

Consider for a moment the general model of a change-process shown in Figure B1. *In general* organizational problems will require *both* analysis *and* the collection of factual data before

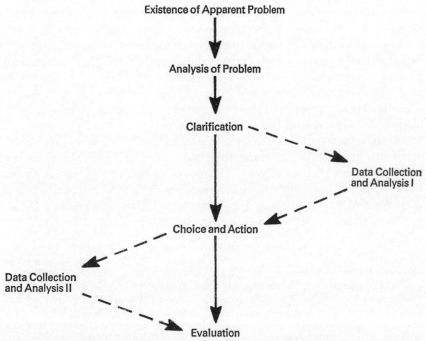

Existence of Apparent Problem

Analysis of Problem

Clarification

Data Collection and Analysis I

Choice and Action

Data Collection and Analysis II

Evaluation

Figure B1   General Model of a Change-Process

rational action can be taken, but the emphasis on the need for analysis of the nature of the problem as opposed to the provision and analysis of factual data, will vary from problem to problem. In social analysis, the assumption is that the problems are such that analysis of their real nature is what is primarily required. For the most part clients are dealing with situations the various facets of which are a matter of direct experience. Where a need for additional factual data does arise, the analyst must either step out of his analytical role and carry out a survey, or must point out to his clients the need for a separate data-collection exercise to be made by some other researcher or member of the organization.[16] Obviously, however, some organizational problems are of quite a different character – the nature of the problem is relatively clear, but what is primarily required is the facts and analysis necessary as a basis for effective action. This might well be the case, for example, in problems of extensive outpatient waiting-time in hospitals, or problems of predicting the demand for beds in various medical specialties.[17]

So too, *in general* it will be possible to strengthen the final process of evaluation of the effectiveness of change in any change-process – whether such an evaluation is made by researcher, client or some third party – with factual data, so that the final judgment may be as informed as possible. Moreover it might be expected that the more necessary and useful the provision of factual or measured data prior to choice of action, the more amenable the situation to providing factual data for evaluation.

In this particular research we are currently heavily occupied with just this problem of the provision of data for evaluation. As the first series of formally sanctioned pilot-projects is about to be launched, we are engaged in designing detailed evaluation procedures and in considering just what significant measures of beneficial change, if any, can possibly be established. We shall be

[16] The latter course has more usually been adopted in the particular social-analytic tradition described here. Indeed there may be acute problems of role-conflict or role-confusion if the analyst tried to do otherwise.

[17] Very often such problems are particularly susceptible to an O.R. (operations research) approach. Indeed it might be predicted that where the *nature* of the problem is already clear and generally agreed so that everybody concerned has a motivation to solve it, an O.R. approach has the highest chances of success; and conversely, that it is most likely to fail where these conditions do not hold.

considering too, the extent to which third parties can contribute to the evaluation process.

Coming back, however, to the initial question of whether change has been achieved so far, and if so, to what extent it is beneficial, the best evidence that can be adduced for the moment is that of cumulative agreements of clients to a range of developing formulations. In general it may be noted that the status of agreement, and hence the feeling of achieved change, will be different at all the various stages shown in Figure B1 above, increasing as the three phases follow one another. To take the extreme case, given some formulation – say of the requisite relationship of chief officer at H.M.C. level (discussed in Chapter 9 above) which had been pilot-tested in one or more individual projects, which had been adopted as general policy by the Regional Authority concerned, and tested wholesale throughout the Region, then the evidence of real and beneficial change would be persuasive, to put it at its mildest.

In fact in the project described here, at the moment of writing, the general state of progress is as follows.

Phase I. Individual Field Projects – Some dozens of field projects have led to agreement by the groups involved of formulations of requisite organizations, in some cases close to what 'exists', in some cases different. Where radical changes are involved a number of these are in process of being sanctioned for pilot test and evaluation, in ways now being designed.

Phase II. Conferences – A number of formulations of hospital organizations as a whole (roughly the range covered in the previous text) have reached some measure of agreement by consensus in multidisciplinary research conference discussions with many hundreds of senior officers. More specific formulations for particular occupational groups are now being tested and agreed in executive conferences.

Phase III. General Organizational Policy Formation – The Regional Board have approved a number of definitions of basic organizational concepts (those listed in Appendix A) for general adoption in executive discussion throughout the Region. They have also approved a statement of the operational activities of the Region (see Chapter 10), and have approved in principle a general statement of the range of possibilities of alternative organizational forms for various parts of the hospital – nursing, medical staff, etc. – roughly the range displayed in Part II.

In effect these various phases of project-work can be thought of as an ever-increasing reinforcement of the processes of change which arise from the first contacts of client and researcher in field project or conference.

Is Social Analysis Scientific?

Finally we come to the question how far, if at all, all this activity could properly be called scientific, or more precisely, to what extent it produces an output of scientific knowledge.

One of the problems in attempting to answer this question is the lack of any general agreement as to what marks genuine scientific method, or more particularly, genuine scientific method in the social sciences. The controversy between those who maintain that social sciences are right to adopt the methods of natural sciences, and those who argue that being *sui generis* they justify valid and different methods of their own, cannot be entered into here.[18] What can be done, at any rate is to note some extremely broad characteristics of a scientific approach over whose validity and importance there would probably be little argument.

(1) The scientist is required to adopt a certain *attitude* in respect to his subject, material or human. The attitude is not necessarily unconcerned, nor is it value-free; but the scientist must never identify completely with his subject, he must always (and obstinately) maintain a degree of critical independence, a certain tough-minded scepticism towards his own hypothesis as well as towards hypothesis of other people.

(2) The stuff of the science itself is *general statements, propositions, theories, models*, framed in *terms* or *concepts* of the sharpest possible definition.[19] The theory must be able to explain the

[18] Bottomore (1971) Chapters 2 and 3 offers a brief introduction to the arguments and principle exponents on each side. Popper (1961) provides a brilliant analysis in depth of the pro-naturalistic and anti-naturalistic arguments.
[19] Toulmin (1953) distinguishes a 'natural-history' approach which collects, records and generalizes a number of observed instances in everyday terms from that of a developed science, in which everyday events are analysed, interpreted, explored in terms of general theories employing newly-created concepts with very special meanings. 'Natural historians, then, look for regularities of given forms; but physicists (sic) seek the form of given regularities' (Chapter II).

reality it mirrors, or at least interpret it; arguably it must be usable to make exact predictions of the outcome in certain combinations of real circumstances.

(3) The theories, models, or whatever, must be *testable*, so that it is possible to make a definite decision as to whether they fit reality as they stand, or whether they need modification to account for reality more adequately.

Using at any rate these rather general characteristics or criteria, let us now examine the extent to which social analysis, as described here, matches up to them.

As far as the first characteristic is concerned, the attempt of the analyst-researcher to maintain a professional detachment at all times, in spite of his commitment to the concern of his client, has already been made. It merely requires to be noted that 'professional detachment' in this context is virtually a synonym for 'scientific attitude'.

Turning to consider the nature of the material actually produced by project-work, it can be seen to consist of statements of four logical classes.

(1) Firstly, these are statements of basic organizational concepts. These cannot be shown to be either right or wrong, but are purely definitional. They are of the form 'the meaning to be assigned to the term x, is y'. For example 'task' which is defined as 'a piece of work with a specific objective which is to be met within some definite time-scale' (Appendix A). The everyday meaning of 'task' bears other definitions. For scientific purposes, one special definition has been assigned.

(2) Secondly, there are statements of more complex organizational concepts or components, often framed in terms of the first definition, for example, the definition of *co-ordinating role*, which employs both the primary concepts of *task* and *authority* in its own definition. These second statements too, are of the form 'the meaning to be assigned to the term x, is y'. Are they, too, purely definitional? They certainly do not make propositions about specific situations, but on the other hand they are modified as they are found adequate or inadequate in describing what is requisite in specific situations. They were described in Chapter 4 in terms of 'packages' of role-properties. Perhaps they are best thought of as basic models, in miniature, of organization, rather than as definitions.

(3) Thirdly, there are statements of what is thought to be requisite

organization as a result of project-work in particular situations, of the form 'in a particular field of work w, in one specific hospital assuming constraints c, the requisite form of organization is x'. These statements employ the basic models of (2). These are the statements, characteristically, that emerge from individual field projects (Phase I).

(4) Fourthly, there are aggregates of these particular statements, which take the form of propositions like 'in particular fields of work w, in all hospitals, assuming constraints c, the following forms x_1, x_2, x_3, etc. are claimed to be requisite'; or, as an alternative formulation 'the following forms of requisite organization x_1, x_2, x_3 etc. must be considered as possibilities'.

So far, these are the only kinds of statements to emerge from project-work. The discussions in conferences, in general reports to the sponsoring authorities, and in this text, go as far as, but no further than, aggregates of possibilities of the form described in (4) above. Very often of course, as in, say, the organizational position of medical consultants, only one organizational form x_1, is thought to be requisite so far, in all hospitals in which we have worked.

However, there seems no reason in principle, why, as project-work in Phase III develops, two further kinds of proposition might not arise and be considered.

(5) Fifthly, there might be empirical generalizations of the form 'organizational models of form x tend to be found requisite in situations of type w, given constraints c'.[20] These would be state-

---

[20] This of course suggests the form of investigation much *à la mode* in current organizational research: for example in Woodward (1965), Lawrence & Lorsch (1967), Pugh et al (1969). To note a minor but important qualification, findings in such research refer to what is requisite rather than what is found *to be* requisite. There are two implications here. Firstly, that the onus is on the researcher rather than the organization member to judge, or set-up measures for what is or is not requisite, i.e. efficient. Or perhaps one should say that it is assumed that both parties use the same criteria in making value-judgments of what is good and what is better. Secondly, there is an implication that data about organizational forms are readily accessible to researchers, and indeed to organization members. Whereas this may be true for certain kinds of data, e.g. numbers of staff employed, it is certainly well worth questioning in the light of this research alone, for other kinds of data, e.g. number of 'supervisory' i.e. managerial, levels in the organization. In other words, it must be questioned very seriously for certain kinds of data, whether the manifest, or assumed, can be equated for survey purposes with either the extant or the requisite.

ments of statistical tendency, and as such could be subject to the usual qualifications on degree of dispersion and degree of significance.

(6) Finally, there might be general theories which attempt to explain *why* a variety of organizational forms x are requisite, in situations of type w under condition c, in terms of more general factors f which determine when and where each of the forms is requisite.

To illustrate generalizations of type (5) above, it might turn out, for example, that there was a tendency for it to be found requisite for nurses in charge to assume managerial control of domestic and catering staff (x) at all hospitals under a certain critical size, and removed more than a certain critical distance from a 'parent' hospital (w) given the present social conditions for recruitment and transport of domestic and catering staff (c). This is a proposition of type (5) though in this case, given the exposition of what is requisite (in the example quoted, in terms of prevailing social arrangements), explanatory theories spring to mind, thus leading immediately to propositions of type (6).

One example of a possible type (6) proposition, is the suggestion that it is never requisite for organization to grow behind one tier of superior-subordinate relationship (x) for any doctor in a clinical situation (w) given the condition that patients are to be in the care of a designated individual doctor, rather than an agency (c), for the reason (f) that such doctors could not take personal responsibility for patients they did not personally see on occasion, and that this regular personal contact in hierarchies of two or more tiers would be tantamount to 'bypassing' of those holding managerial roles at intermediate levels (see Chapter 5).

It seems then that the process of social analysis does, or in some cases might readily, produce a whole range of conceptual definitions and theoretical propositions of the form to be expected in any scientific enquiry. This still leaves the last and crucial question: in what way are these propositions testable?

Since propositions of type (5) refer factually to what tends to be 'found' (i.e. believed, claimed) requisite in a number of similar situations, they may of course, be tested by applying the normal measures of statistical tendency and significance. Again, propositions of type (4) are not in this sense a separate category – they are a half step as it were from type (3) to type (5) propositions. As they stand, their validity entirely rests on the validity of the individual type (3) propositions from which they are compared. So we are left with type (3) and type (5) propositions, and here all turns in the end on demonstrating that some or other organizational arrangement is in fact 'requisite'. Since the whole process of analysis and test turns on this key-notion, it behoves to consider it yet again.

What is the requisite? It is in other language, the most *efficient* answer, the most *productive* answer, the *optimum* answer;[21] in short the best answer to any given problem given *certain prescribed constraints* and *conditions*.[22] But who is to judge efficiency, who is to judge requisiteness? Here we are back to the great divide and it is, of course, the same divide as was reached in pursuing (in the previous section) the question of the extent of useful change achieved. There the question appeared as 'who is to judge

[21] Or rather than the optimum, the requisite is in the words of March & Simon (1958) that which is found *satisfactory* in any decision-making situation, in relation to the time and effort that can be devoted to exploring reasonable possibilities, as opposed to what in a more theoretical sense, might be 'optimum'.

[22] Alternatively, again, one might describe it as the *functional* or *most functional* answer, thus drawing attention here to certain similarities in outlook to that of a major sociological school – Durkheim, Radcliffe-Brown, Malinowski, Merton etc. (see for example Merton, 1968). However a crucial difference must be noted between 'functionalism' as teleological explanation in 'pure' research, on the one hand, and the study of function in applied research as in this project, on the other, where the question posed is to do with 'how functional' are various alternative forms for certain ends which are already given.

A common criticism of the functional mode of analysis in pure sociology is its tendency to justify the extant in all situations and to underplay the importance of social conflict and social change. This criticism of 'functionalism' does not appear to be so valid in the applied research method described here, which takes every account of social conflict and is simply dedicated to social change! The spirit is in essence that of 'piecemeal social engineering' (Popper 1957) where the 'social engineer' designs social institutions which are 'functional' or 'instrumental' in meeting the end desired by those with whom he works.

In many ways the approach is an 'action' one rather than functionalist (Silverman 1970). The divergent definitions of the situation of the various actors in it are freely accepted as a usual starting point, although the aim is to reach consensus on what is functional assuming the presence of some 'central value system' as Parsons calls it, which allows such work to be undertaken.

if change is beneficial?' Here, it reappears as 'who is to judge if change is requisite?' Again, the questions must be separated, on the one hand, of the extent and validity of any factual data that may significably be brought to bear, and, on the other, of who it is makes the ultimate value judgment. We would maintain that the question of efficiency or requisiteness in human affairs must always in the end be a matter of value judgment, however comprehensive the relevant data. It is possible to argue that none are better equipped to perform this crucial test than those who are affected by its consequences, i.e. the organization members who collaborate in the science-seeking-cum-change-seeking process: or one may argue on the contrary that only a third party can make a 'really objective' judgment of whether efficiency has or has not increased.

The more pressing problem at this stage is, as we have said before, to discover what measures if any, really will help to facilitate the evacuation of projects, and if there are any, to get them established in use[23]. Although it is undoubtedly hoped that any changes will in the long run be to the benefit of the performance of the hospital as a whole, it seems clear that there are far too many intervening variables to allow measures of things such as length of stay by patients, staff turnover, or direct clinical evaluations of care of patients,[24] to be regarded as significant indications of beneficial change. The focus for the moment must be on ways of getting significant data on the improvement in personal working relationships between those directly affected by redefinitions or clarifications of role, or others indirectly affected.[25]

In considering social analysis as a scientific process, one further aspect bears comment. This, however, is an aspect of no mean importance.

One of the great problems of all social research (though it is in fact equally a feature of research in the natural sciences) is to deal

[23] As Weiland (1971, page 219) points out, one of the problems with action-research, in hospitals as elsewhere, is to know what variables to measure before and after the change, when the exact directions of activity are still to be defined.

[24] See definition in Georgopoulos and Mann, 1962, Chapter 5.

[25] Some of the general problems of making adequate and significant assessments of organizational change are sensitively traced by Sofer (1963). He draws attention particularly to dangers in the too-ready use of 'productivity' measures.

with the interaction-effect of the researcher on his subject. Ideally it seems that the researcher wants to get 'objective' knowledge of behaviour or characteristics of his subject; but in the very act of observing, he interacts with his subject, and his subjects react in turn, modifying their behaviour or character to some degree or other, and thus detracting from the objectivity of the observation. The problem, conceived as one of reducing random disturbances in social experiments, has long been recognized. More recent writers (for example, Rosenthal 1966, Friedman 1967) have suggested that something rather more radical than a 'random-disturbance' is in evidence here.

Social analysis meets this situation in an interesting way, making as it were, a virtue of necessity. The interaction is not minimized, in fact it becomes a central feature of the proceedings. Knowledge is not thought of as being there to be had, to be collected at will; knowledge is there to be created, to be hewn with effort from rough and ill-shaped starting materials. 'Valid' knowledge is the hard-won understanding of what really is and what really works, which must be obtained by change agent and client in close collaboration. However, a warning is necessary: collaboration, if conceived simply as a honey-sweet process of co-operation is too naïve a concept here. In an effective passage (pages 147-153) Bennis, Benne & Chin illuminate the relation of collaboration and conflict in the field and conclude:

(1) Collaboration is an achievement not a given condition. The ways of effective collaboration must be learned.

(2) Conflict is not to be avoided by a change agent, he faces conflicts in himself and in others and seeks ways to channel the energies of conflict towards the achievement of personal and social gain for all concerned.

(3) Power is not a bad thing, though much behavioural science literature treats it as such through indifference or ignorance.

(4) Social action depends on power just as physical movement depends on energy. Nothing changes in human affairs until new power is generated or until old power is redistributed.

(5) The change agent strives to utilize power that is based on and guided by rationality, valid knowledge, and collaboration and to discount power based on and channelled by fear, irrationality, and coercion. The latter kind of power leads to augumented resistance to change, unstable changes, and dehumanized and irrational conflicts.

Bibliography

Note: Government reports are listed under the Department of origin (e.g. 'Ministry of Health') and cross-referenced to the commonly-used identification (e.g. 'Salmon' 'Cogwheel').

ABEL-SMITH, B. (1964), *The Hospitals 1800–1948*, London: Heinemann.

ACTON SOCIETY TRUST (1955), *Hospitals and the State: Hospital Organization and Administration Under the National Health Service, Vols. 1-6*, London, Acton Society Trust.

ANDERSON, J. A. D. et al (1971), 'Consultants' Role in Hospital Management', *The Medical Officer*, 125, Part 6, pp. 73-77.

ARGYRIS, C. (1964), *Integrating the Individual and the Organisation*, London: Wiley.

BALES, R. F. (1966), 'Task Roles and Social Roles in Problem-Solving Groups' in BIDDLE, B. J. and THOMAS, E. J. (1966) (eds.), op. cit.

BENNIS, W. G., BENNE, K. D. and CHIN, R. (1970), *The Planning of Change*, 2nd edn., London: Holt, Rinehart and Winston.

BERGER, J. (1969), *A Fortunate Man, The Story of a Country Doctor*, Harmondsworth: Penguin.

BIDDLE, B. J. and THOMAS, E. J. (eds.) (1966), *Role Theory: Concepts and Research*, London: Wiley.

BLAKE, R. R. and MOUTON, J. S. (1964), *The Managerial Grid*, Houston: Gulf Publishing Company.

BLAU, P. M. and SCOTT, W. R. (1964), *Formal Organisations*, London: Routledge & Kegan Paul.

BOTTOMORE, T. B. (1971), *Sociology, A Guide to the Problems and Literature*, 2nd Edn., London: Allen & Unwin.

BRADBEER REPORT (1954) – see MINISTRY OF HEALTH (1954).

BRADFORD, L. P., GIBB, J. R. and BENNE, K. D. (Eds.) (1964), *Group Theory and Laboratory Method*, New York: Wiley.

BROTHERSTON REPORT (1967) – see SCOTTISH HOME AND HEALTH DEPARTMENT (1967).

BROWN, W. (1960), *Exploration in Management*, London: Heinemann.

BROWN, W. (1971), *Organization*, London: Heinemann.

BROWN, W. and JAQUES, E. (1965), *Glacier Project Papers*, London: Heinemann.

CENTRAL MIDWIVES BOARD (1962), *Handbook Incorporating the Rules of the Central Midwives Board*, 25th edn., London: Central Midwives Board.

CENTRAL OFFICE OF INFORMATION (1968), *Health Services in Britain*, London: H.M.S.O.

CHAPLIN, N. W. (1969), 'The National Health Service' in MILNE, T. F. and CHAPLIN, N. W. *Modern Hospital Management*, London: Institute of Hospital Administration.

'COGWHEEL' REPORT (1967) – see MINISTRY OF HEALTH (1967).

COOPER, E. J. (1971), 'Beyond Functional Management', *Hospital*, 67 (5), pp. 158-163.

CORNISH, J. B. (1971), 'Research and the Management of Hospitals' in MCLACHLAN (ed.) (1971), op. cit.

CORNISH, J. B. and MACDONALD, A. G. (1971), 'Operational Research' in MCLACHLAN, G. (ed.) (1971), op. cit.

CRICHTON, A. and HARDIE, R. (1965), *The Need for Manpower Planning in the Hospital Service*, Welsh Hospital Staff Committee, Welsh Hospital Board.

DALE, E. and URWICK, L. F. (1960), *Staff in Organisations*, New York: McGraw Hill.

DEPARTMENT OF HEALTH AND SOCIAL SECURITY (1968), *Hospital Scientific & Technical Services* (Zuckerman), London: H.M.S.O.

DEPARTMENT OF HEALTH AND SOCIAL SECURITY (1968), *Relieving Nurses of Non-Nursing Duties in General and Maternity Hospitals* (Farrer), London: H.M.S.O.

DEPARTMENT OF HEALTH AND SOCIAL SECURITY (1969), *The Functions of the District General Hospital* (Bonham-Carter), London: H.M.S.O.

DEPARTMENT OF HEALTH AND SOCIAL SECURITY (1969), *Report of the Committee of Inquiry into Allegations of Ill-Treatment of Patients and other irregularities at the Ely Hospital, Cardiff*, Cmnd. 3970. London: H.M.S.O.

DEPARTMENT OF HEALTH AND SOCIAL SECURITY (1969), *The Responsibilities of the Consultant Grade* (Godber), London: H.M.S.O.

DEPARTMENT OF HEALTH AND SOCIAL SECURITY (1970), *Report of the Working Party on the Hospital Pharmaceutical Service* (Noel-Hall), London: H.M.S.O.

DEPARTMENT OF HEALTH AND SOCIAL SECURITY (1970), *The Future Structure of the National Health Service* (Second Green Paper), London: H.M.S.O.

DEPARTMENT OF HEALTH AND SOCIAL SECURITY (1970), *Hospital Building Maintenance* (Woodbine-Parish), London: H.M.S.O.

DEPARTMENT OF HEALTH AND SOCIAL SECURITY (1971), *Report of the Farleigh Hospital Committee of Enquiry*, Cmnd. 4557, London: H.M.S.O.

DEPARTMENT OF HEALTH AND SOCIAL SECURITY (1971), *National Health Service: Consultation Document*, (Limited Circulation).

ELY REPORT (1969) – see DEPARTMENT OF HEALTH AND SOCIAL SECURITY (1969).

ETZIONI, A. (1964), *Modern Organisations*, Englewood Cliffs, N. J.: Prentice-Hall.

ETZIONI, A. (ed.) (1969), *The Semi-Professions and Their Organisation*, New York: The Free Press.

EVANS, J. (1970), *Managerial Accountability, Chief Officers, Consultants and*

Boards, (unpublished paper) School of Social Sciences, Brunel University.

FARLEIGH REPORT (1971) – see DEPARTMENT OF HEALTH AND SOCIAL SECURITY (1971).

FARQUHARSON-LANG REPORT (1966) – see SCOTTISH HOME AND HEALTH DEPARTMENT (1966).

FARRER REPORT (1968) – see DEPARTMENT OF HEALTH AND SOCIAL SECURITY (1968).

FIEDLER, F. E. (1966), *A Theory of Leadership Effectiveness*, New York: McGraw-Hill.

FREIDSON, E. (Ed.) (1963), *The Hospital in Modern Society*, New York: The Free Press.

FREIDSON, E .(1970), *Professional Dominance: The Social Structure of Medical Care*, New York: Atherton Press.

FRIEDMAN, N. (1967), *The Social Nature of Psychological Research*, New York: Basic Books.

GEORGOPOULOS, F. S. and MANN, F. C. (1962), *The Community General Hospital*, New York: Macmillan.

GERTH, H. H. and MILLS, C. W. (1948), *From Max Weber*, London: Routledge & Kegan Paul.

GODBER REPORT (1969) – see DEPARTMENT OF HEALTH (1969).

GOFFMAN, E. (1968), *Asylums*, London: Penguin Books.

GOODE, W. J. (1969), 'The Theoretical Limits of Professionalisation' in ETZIONI (ed.) (1969), op. cit.

GOODE, W. J. and HATT, P. K. (1953), *Methods in Social Research*, New York: McGraw Hill.

GOSS, M. F. W. (1963), 'Patterns of Bureaucracy among Hospital Staff Physicians' in FREIDSON, E. (ed.) (1963), op. cit.

GOWER, L. C. B. (1957), *Principles of Modern Company Law*, 2nd Edn., London: Stevens.

GRIFFITH, J. A. G. (1966), *Central Departments and Local Authorities*, London: Allen & Unwin.

GROSS, E. (1969), 'The Definition of Organisational Goals', *Brit. J. Sociol.*, 220, pp. 277-294.

GROSS, N., MASON, W. S. and MCEACHERN, A. W. (1957), *Exploration in Role Analysis: Studies of the School Superintendency Role*, New York: Wiley.

GUILLEBAUD REPORT (1956) – see MINISTRY OF HEALTH 1956.

GULICK, L. and URWICK, L. (1937), *Papers on the Science of Administration*, New York: Columbia University.

HOME OFFICE et al (1968), *Report of the Committee on Local Authority and Allied Public Services* (Seebohm), Cmnd. 3703, London: H.M.S.O.

HUMBLE, J. W. (1970), *Management by Objectives in Action*, London: McGraw-Hill.

HUNT REPORT (1966) – see MINISTRY OF HEALTH (1966).

HUNTER, T. D. (1967), 'Hierarchy or Arena?' The Administrative Implications of a Sociotherapeutic Regime, in H. FREEMAN and J. FARNDALE (Eds.) *New Aspects of the Mental Health Service*, Oxford. Pergamon.

JACKSON, J. A. (ed.) (1970), *Professions and Professionalisation*, London: Cambridge U.P.

JACKSON, J. M. (1966), 'Structural Characteristics of Norms' in BIDDLE and THOMAS (eds.) (1966), op. cit.

JAQUES, E. (1951), *The Changing Culture of a Factory*, London: Tavistock Publications.

JAQUES, E. (1956), *Measurement of Responsibility*, London: Heinemann.

JAQUES, E. (1967), *Equitable Payment*, 2nd edn., Harmondsworth: Penguin.

KATZ, D. and KAHN, R. L. (1966), *The Social Psychology of Organisations*, New York: Wiley.

KING EDWARD'S HOSPITAL FUND (1967), *The Shape of Hospital Management in 1980?* (Report of a Joint Working Party of the King's Fund and I.H.A.), London: King Edward's Hospital Fund.

KOGAN, M., CANG, S., DIXON, M. and TOLLIDAY, H. (1971), *Working Relationships Within the British Hospital Service*, London: Bookstall Publications.

LAWRENCE, P. R., and LORSCH, J. W. (1967), *Organization and Environment*, Boston: Harvard University Press.

LIKERT, R. (1961), *New Patterns of Management*, New York: McGraw-Hill.

MCGREGOR, D. (1960), *The Human Side of Enterprise*, New York: McGraw-Hill.

MCLACHLAN, G. (ed.) (1971), *Portfolio for Health, The Role and Programme of the D.H.S.S. in Health Services Research*, Problems and Progress in Medical Care, Sixth Series, London: Oxford U.P.

MAUD REPORT (1967) – see MINISTRY OF HOUSING AND LOCAL GOVERNMENT (1967).

MARCH, J. G. (ed.) (1965), *Handbook of Organisations*, Chicago: Rand McNally.

MARCH, J. G. and SIMON, H. A. (1958), *Organizations*, New York: Wiley.

MENZIES, I .E. P. (1960), 'A Case-Study in the Functioning of Social Systems as a Defence against Anxiety – A Report on a Study of the Nursing Service of a General Hospital', *Human Relations* 13, pp. 93-120.

MERTON, R. K. (1968), *Social Theory and Social Structure*, (3rd Edn.), New York: Free Press.

MERTON, R. K., READER, G. G. and KENDALL, P. L. (eds.) (1957), *The Student-Physician*, Cambridge, Mass.: Harvard U.P.

MILES, A. W. and SMITH, D. (1969), *Joint Consultation, Defeat or Opportunity?* London: King Edward's Hospital Fund.

MILLER, E. J. and RICE, A. K. (1967), *Systems of Organisation*, London: Tavistock Publications.

MINISTRY OF HEALTH (1954), *Report of the Committee on Internal Administration of Hospitals* (Bradbeer), London: H.M.S.O.

MINISTRY OF HEALTH (1956), *Report of the Committee of Enquiry into the Cost of the National Health Service* (Guillebaud), Cmnd. 9663, London: H.M.S.O.

MINISTRY OF HEALTH (1961), *Medical Staffing Structure in the Hospital Service* (Platt), London: H.M.S.O.

MINISTRY OF HEALTH (1962), *A Hospital Plan for England and Wales*, Cmnd. 1604, London: H.M.S.O.

MINISTRY OF HEALTH (1966), *Report of the Committee on Hospital Supplies Organisation* (Hunt), London: H.M.S.O.

MINISTRY OF HEALTH (1966), Report of the Committee on Senior Nursing Staff Structure (Salmon), London: H.M.S.O.

MINISTRY OF HEALTH (1967), *First Report of the Joint Working Party on the Organisation of Medical Work in Hospitals* (Godber – The 'Cogwheel' Report), London: H.M.S.O.

MINISTRY OF HEALTH (1968), *National Health Service: The Administrative Structure of the Medical and Related Services in England and Wales* (First Green Paper), London: H.M.S.O.

MINISTRY OF HOUSING AND LOCAL GOVERNMENT (1967), *Management of Local Government* (Volume 1) (Maud), London: H.M.S.O.

MOUZELIS, N. P. (1967), *Organisation and Bureaucracy*, London: Routledge & Kegan Paul.

NADEL, S. F. (1957), *The Theory of Social Structure*, London: Cohen and West.

NAYLOR, W. M. (1971), *Organisation and Management of a Unified Health Service: Organisation of Area Health Services*, London: Institute of Health Service Administrators.

NEWMAN, A. D. and ROWBOTTOM, R. W. (1968), *Organization Analysis*, London: Heinemann.

NOEL-HALL REPORT (1970) – see DEPARTMENT OF HEALTH AND SOCIAL SECURITY (1970).

NURSING TIMES (1969), 'Ward Housekeeping' Two Occasional Papers, 4th and 11th December 1969.

OWEN, A. H. (1971), 'The Relationships between Central and Local Authorities', *Public Administration*, 49, pp. 439-456.

PACKWOOD, G. F. L. (1971), 'The Role of Deputy in the Hospital Service' in *The Hospital*, 67, pp. 271-275.

PANTALL, J. and ELLIOTT, J. (1968), *Can Research Aid Hospital Management*, London: The Hospital Centre (Reprint 234).

PARSONS, T. (1951), *The Social System*, London: Routledge & Kegan Paul.

PERROW, C. (1965), 'Hospitals: Technology, Structure and Goals', in MARCH, J. A. (ed.) op. cit.

PERROW, C. (1970), *Organizational Analysis, A Sociological View*, London: Tavistock.

PLATT REPORT (1961) – see MINISTRY OF HEALTH (1961).

POPPER, K. R. (1960), *The Poverty of Historicism*, 2nd edn., London: Routledge & Kegan Paul.

PUGH, D. S., HICKSON, D. J., HININGS, C. R. and TURNER, C. (1969), 'The Context of Organisation Structures', *Administrative Science Quarterly*, 14, (i), pp. 91-114.

READER, L. G. (1963), 'Contributions of Sociology to Medicine' in FREEMAN, H. E. and LEVINE, L. G. (eds.), *Handbook of Medical Sociology*, Englewood Cliffs, N.J.: Prentice-Hall.

REDDIN, W. T. (1970), *Managerial Effectiveness*, New York: McGraw-Hill.

REVANS, R. W. (1964), *Standards for Morale; Cause and Effect in Hospitals*, London: Oxford University Press.

REVANS, R. W. (ed.) (1971) (In Press), *Hospitals: Communications, Choice and Change*, London: Tavistock

RICHARDSON, R. (1971), *Fair Pay and Work*, London: Heinemann.

ROETHLISBERGER, F. J. and DICKSON, W. J. (1939), *Management and the Worker*, Cambridge. Mass.: Harvard U.P.

ROSEN, G. (1963), 'The Hospital – Historical Sociology of a Community Institution' in FREIDSON, E. (ed.) (1963), op. cit.

ROSENTHAL, R. (1966), *Experimenter Effects in Behavioural Research*, New York: Appleton-Century Crofts.

ROWBOTTOM, R. W. and HEY, A. M., 'Towards an Organisation of Social Service Departments' (1970), *Local Government Chronicle*, 5403, p. 1849.

SALMON REPORT (1966) – see MINISTRY OF HEALTH (1966)

SCOTTISH HOME AND HEALTH DEPARTMENT (1966), *Administrative Practice of Hospital Boards in Scotland* (Farquharson-Lang), Edinburgh: H.M.S.O.

SCOTTISH HOME AND HEALTH DEPARTMENT (1967), *Organisation of Medical Work in the Hospital Service in Scotland* (Brotherston), Edinburgh: H.M.S.O.

SEEBOHM REPORT (1968) – see HOME OFFICE (1968).

SILVERMAN, D. (1970), *The Theory of Organisation*, London: Heinemann.

SIMON, H. A. (1957), *Administrative Behaviour*, New York: Macmillan.

SOFER, C. (1964), 'The Assessment of Organisational Change', *Journal of Management Studies*, 1, 128-142.

SLEIGHT, P., SPENCER, J. A. and TOWLER, E. W. (1970), 'Oxford and McKinsey: Cogwheel and Beyond', *Brit Med. J.*, 1, 682-684.

SMITH, H. L. (1958), 'Two Lines of Authority: The Hospital's Dilemma' in JACO, E. G. (ed.) *Patients, Physicians and Illness, Source Book in Behavioural Science and Medicine*, Glencoe Ill.: Free Press.

STANTON, A. H. and SCHWARTZ, M. S. (1954), *The Mental Hospital*, New York: Basic Books.

STEWART, R. and SLEEMAN, J. (1967), *Continuously Under Review, A Study of the Management of Outpatient Departments*, Occasional Papers in Social Administration, No. 20. London: Bell.

STINCHCOMBE, A. L. (1965), 'Social Structure and the Invention of Organisational Forms' in MARCH, J. A. (ed.) (1965), op. cit.

STUART-CLARK, A. C. (1956), *Administering the Hospital Group, The Work of the Management Committee Member*, London: Institute of Hospital Administrators.

TOULMIN, S. (1953), *The Philosophy of Science*, London: Heinemann.

WEILAND, G. F. and LEIGH, H. E. (eds.) (1971), *Changing Hospitals: A Report on the H.I.C. Project*. London: Tavistock.

WILLIAMS, D. (1969), 'The Administrative Contribution of the Nursing Sister', *Public Administration*, Autumn, 307-28.

WOODBINE-PARISH REPORT (1970) – see DEPARTMENT OF HEALTH AND SOCIAL SECURITY (1970).

WOODWARD, J. (1965), *Industrial Organization: Theory and Practice*, London: Oxford University Press.

ZUCKERMAN REPORT (1968) – see DEPARTMENT OF HEALTH AND SOCIAL SECURITY (1968).

Index

ABEL SMITH, B., 148 234
Accident and emergency department, 137
Accountability, 30, 31, 37, 261
  to fellow professionals, 78
  to patients, 78
Acting management, deputizing and, 265
'Acting-up', 57
Acton Society Trust Survey of Hospitals, 14
Administration, medical and medical representation
  relationship with heads of departments and officers, 98, 151, 152
Administrative, Medical Officer of Region, Senior, 81
  organization, Group, 180, 181, 182
  staff, and consultants, 84
  functional and geographical organization, 180-7
  relationship to hospital doctor, 89-90
Administrator, Chief, authority in respect of Treasurer, 184, 185
  role of, 173-7
Administrators, and paramedical work, 102, 103
Allocation officer (nursing), 134, 136
Analysis, social, see social analysis
Analysts social, 294-300
Analytic relationship, limit of, 281
Anderson, J. A. D., et al, 74
Appeals or grievance procedures, 261
Area Health Authority, 51
Argyris, C., 32
Assessment, 261
Assistants, role of, 56, 59
Assumed situation, 4
Attachment, 62, 262

dual influence situation, 221
  relationship of ward housekeeper, 165
Audiology technicians, 101
Authority, 263, 295
Autonomy, clinical and professional, 74, 75, 214-18

BALES, R. F., 68
Berger, J., 79
Bennis, W. G. et al, 288
Biddle, B. J. et al, 36
Biochemist, Principal in relation to Chief Pathologist, 86
  organizational position of, 113, 114
  role of, 101
  work of, 108
Blake, R. R. et al, 67
Blau, P. M. et al, 6
Boards of Governors, 9, 15, 21, 80, 93, 99, 175
Bonham-Carter Report, 20
Bottomore, T. B., 294
Bradbeer Report, 13, 47, 99, 186, 206, 238
Bradford, L. P. et al, 282
Brotherston Report, 98
Brown, W., 25, 38, 40, 46, 57, 130, 248, 258, 279
  and Jaques, E., 37, 43, 130, 277, 281
Brunel University, School of Social Sciences, 1
Budgets and programmes (engineering and building), 159
Builders, 56, 100, 196
'Building blocks' of requisite organization, 260
Building, and engineering work, nature of, 159

Building, and engineering—*Cont.*
    organization of, 151, 152
    foreman, supervisory role of, 150
    maintenance and development, 179
    officers, 151
        regional, 148
    Supervisor, 152, 158, 206
Bureaucratic organization, 96, 97

C.S.S.D. (Central Sterile Supplies
    Department), 149
Cang, S., 41
Cardiological technicians, 113
Caterers, 100, 196
Catering, manager, 123
    services, 169, 173
    staff, relationships with, 123
Central, Government, influence of, 253
    Middlesex Group, 2
    Sterile Supplies Department, *see*
        C.S.S.D.
Chairman, elected, 93, 94
    of the Board of Governors, 21
    of Governing Body, 21, 252
    of H.M.C., 20
    of Medical Committees, 86
Change agent, 289
    processes, 288-94
Chaplin, N. W., 15
Charing Cross Group, London, 1
Chief Nursing Officer, 131, 138, 144,
        202, 203, 206
    relationship to Allocation Officer, 142,
        143
    relationship to nurse in charge of
        small hospital, 144
    relationship to P.N.O., 131, 143
    see also Group C.N.O. and Regional
        C.N.O.
Chief Officers, function of in control of
        expenditure, 182-7, 237
Chiropodists, 101, 114
Cleaners, 120, 122, 177, 196
Clerical staff in pathology complex, 107
Clinical assistants, 87
    autonomy, 94
    research and teaching, provision for,
        193, 196
Coalition or collegiate role-structure in
        hospitals, 65
'Cogwheel', 13, 75, 98, 230, 238 (*see also*
        Godber)

Collaboration, 2, 3, 277, 278
    and conflict, 300
    unstructured, 226
Collateral relationship, 52, 53, 54, 263
Collegiate structure, 65, 85, 87, 256, 263
Co-management, *see* Attachment
Committee (True), 65, 263
Community Development Project
        (Brunel), 213
Conference, executive, 284
    research, 283
    training, 284
Conferences, aims of, 1
Conflict and collaboration, 300
Consultant, basic duties of, 75
    definition of, 98
    paediatrician, 54
    staff, clinical autonomy of, 75, 84
Consultants, relationship to, each other,
        85
    general practitioner, 90
    junior medical staff, 85
    nursing staff, 88
    R.H.B. or Board of Governors, 80
Consultative Councils, *see* Joint Con-
        sultative Councils
Contracts of employment of consultants,
        termination of, 78
Cooper, E. J., 177
Co-ordinated group, multiple manage-
        ment, 219
Co-ordinating, and monitoring function
        of Group Secretary, 173-7
    relationship, 47-9
    role, 264
    see also Monitoring and co-ordinating
Co-ordination, in health organization,
        problems of, 223, 225
    of medical work, 229, 230
Cornish, J. B., 12, 13
Cottage hospitals, 21
    consultant relationship, 90
    G.P. facilities, 90
    see also General Practitioner Hospitals
Crichton, A. et al, 12
Cross-over point, 53, 55, 90, 265
Cytology, clinical assistant, 107

D.H.S.S. (Department of Health and
        Social Security), 1, 3, 9
    Circular (71) 82, 114

D.H.S.S.—*Cont.*
N.H.S. Reorganization Consultative
document, 251
H.M. (70) 17, 257
Dale, E. et al, 248
Day nurseries, 18
Decision making, 250, 251, 252
Dental staff, 18
Dentists, 16, 17
Department, of Health and Social
Security, *see* D.H.S.S.
head, relationship to hospital organ-
ization, 150-2
Deputies, 56, 57, 59
Deputizing and acting management,
265, 266
Dietetics, 153
Dietitians, 101, 102, 114, 120
Dispensing opticians, 16
District general hospital, 20
Dixon, N., 41
Doctor, and his patient, 78
monitoring work of, 215
Doctors, in hospital, 6, 16, 96, 97, 102,
120
organizational position of, 7
junior, 178
Domestic, organization, 59, 150, 151,
163-9
Dual-influence situations, 59, 221
hospital head of department, 154
supplies officer, 161
Dulwich Hospital Housekeeping Pro-
ject, 10, 164
Durkheim, 298
Duties, 266
Duty, 37

EAST BIRMINGHAM HOSPITAL GROUP, 4
Elliott, J. *see* Pantall, J.
Ely Report, 31, 198, 207, 208
Engineer, Group, 8, 19, 148, 202-5
Regional, relationship to Group
Engineer, 202-5
Engineering and building, 151, 152,
158-61
Etzioni, A., 35, 96, 117, 231
Evans, J., 80
Executive, Committee, United Oxford
Hospitals, 244
councils, 16

conference, 284
hierarchy, 65, 266
system, 266
Expenditure, control of, 186, 187
Extant, situation, 46, 14, 35, 267
in Pathology complex, 107
see also Manifest

FAMILY PRACTITIONER SERVICES, 16
Farleigh report, 31, 207
Farquharson-Lang report, 13, 20, 183,
186, 235, 249
Farrer Report, 119, 146, 163, 164
Felt-fair pay, 37
Fiedler, F. E., 67
Finance staff, 196
Financial, Officer, Chief, 183-7
work, 247
see also Treasurer
Freidson, E., 73, 78, 80, 97, 215, 218
Friedman, N., 300
Functional, answer, 37
monitoring and co-ordinating, 60, 62,
81, 205

G.M.C. DISCIPLINARY COMMITTEE, 77
General Medical Council, *see* G.M.C.
G.P., beds, 91, 92
relationship to nurse in charge of
small hospital, 145
G.P.s and Hospital Medical Staff Com-
mittee, 236
General Practitioner Hospitals, 21, 90-2
Georgopoulos, F. S. et al, 299
Geriatric cases, planning of services, 227
Glacier Project, 25, 37, 38, 40, 43, 46,
57, 248, 277, 281, 282
Glacier Metal Co., 130, 258
Godber Report (Cogwheel), 13, 98
see also Cogwheel
Goffman, E., 6
Goode, W. J., 97, 287
Goss, N. et al, 13, 87, 91, 96
Gouldner, 87
Governing body, *see* Regional Hospital
Board and Board of Governors
Gower, L. C. B., 184
Grievance, procedures, *see* Appeals or
grievance procedures
systems, review and, 257, 258
Griffith, J. A. G., 253
Gross, E., 34, 36

Group administration, 182-3
  advisers at hospital level, 156-8
  Chief Administrator, relationship to,
    Group head of department, 150
    Group suplies officer, 152   p
  role of, 173-7
  Chief Nursing Officer, 3, 8, 20
  see also Chief Nursing Officer
  Heads of Departments, 154-7
  and hospital level, Organization at,
    153-6
  Secretary, 3, 6, 20, 82, 173-7
Guillebaud Report, 14, 20, 208, 238
Gulick, L. et al, 247

HAEMATOLOGIST, consultant, 86, 108
Health, Ministry of, see D.H.S.S.
  Authority, 255, 256
    Services, integration of, 244, 245
  organization, problems of, 223, 224
  services, 15, 16
Hierarchical organization, 103, 224, 227
Hierarchy, 68, 93, 252
  and bureaucracy, 68, 69
  executive, 65, 266
  managerial characteristics of, 93
Hillingdon Hospital Group, 2
Histology, consultant in, 86, 107
Hospital, Administrators, Institute of,
    see Insitute of Hospital Adminis-
    trators
  building and maintenance, Wood-
    bine-Parish report, 148, 158
  Centre in Nursing Establishment, see
    Joint Working Party
  facilities, basic in a Unified Health
    Service, 191
  Group Steering Committees, 3
  Internal Communications Project, 3,
    4, 12, 286, 289
  Management, Committee, 8, 19, 51,
    81-4, 110, 172, 173
  shape of in 1980, see King Edward's
    Hospital Fund Report
  Organization Research Unit (Brunel),
    1, 213
  Secretaries, 177, 178, 179
  Service, role of doctors as a group, 73,
    74, 75
  Service, operational activities of,
    definition, 191-3
  scientific and technical staff, 100

Hospitals, staff roles in, 58
'Hotel services' in hospitals, 149
House Committee, 20
Housekeepers, see Domestic organiza-
    tion
  Senior, 167
Housekeeping, projects, 164-9
  staff, organization of, 163-7
  teams, roles and relationships, 163-7
  Supervisors, see Domestic Supervisors
House-surgeon, relationship to consult-
    ant, 87
Humble, J. W., 37
Hunt Report on Hospital-Supplies
    Organization, 148, 152, 161
Hunter, T. D., 68

INDIVIDUAL ROLE, 27
Institute of Hospital Administrators,
    197
Institutional services, 234-9

JAQUES, E., 25, 32, 37, 170, 277, 280,
    281, 282
Joint, Consultative Councils, 64
  Working Party Report of the Royal
    College of Nursing and the
    National Council of Nurses and
    the Hospital Centre on Nursing
    Establishment, 146

KATZ, D. et al, 34, 282
Kendall, 225
King Edward's College, London, 1
King Edward's Hospital Fund Report,
    235
Kitchen Superintendents, role of, 150
Kogan, M. et al, 41, 222

LABORATORY TECHNICIANS, 101
Langdon-Davies, see Abel Smith, B.
Laundry, staff, 54
  and linen services, 148, 150, 151, 169
  and linen staff, 149
Lawrence, P. R. et al, 67, 177, 296
Level-of-work, 37
Lewins, K., 288
Likert, R., 67
Linen services, see Laundry and linen
    services

Lippit, et al, 288
Local, authority, 17, 18
    authority, Social Services Act 1970, 18
    social worker, 54
    Dental Committee, 17
    Health Committees, 17
    Health Services, 17, 18
    Medical Committee, 17
    Medical Committee, Chairman of, on
        H.M.C., 199
    Social Service Committee, 18

MCGREGOR, 67
McKinsay Management Consultants, 244
Malinowski, 298
Management, deputizing and acting, 265
    functional, 221
    systems, unified and multiple, 218
Managerial, hierarchy, 93, 266
    role, of hospital doctors, 280
        in nursing, 132, 133
        natural, 137
    style, 67
    type of work, 247
Manager/subordinate relationship, 42
    see also Superior-subordinate rela-
        tionship
Manifest, organization of Maternity
        Division, 135
    situation, 4, 35, 267, 279
    structure, 14
March, J. G. et al, 298
Maternity, Case services for, 227
    liaison committees, 229
    division, project in, 133, 134, 135
Matron, 206
    relationship to Domestic Superintend-
        ent, 163
Maud Report, 249
Medical, Administration, and medical
        representation, 98
    Administrator, administrative duties
        of, 82
    assistants, relationship to consultants,
        87
    Committee, Chairman of, 82
    committees, role of, 7, 207
    organization, 73-99
    photographers, 114, 101
    Practices Committee, 16
    records, 170, 171, 173
        Officer, Group, 156

    organization of, 149, 151, 153
    register, removal from, 77
    secretarial staff, 54
    secretariat, organization of, 149, 151,
        170, 171
    social, work,
        workers, 101, 114
    staff, committee, 199
        relation of Group Secretary to, 176,
            177
    Superintendent, 82, 95
Menzies, I. E. P., 12
Merit payments (to consultants), 81
Merton, R. K. et al, 78, 225, 298
Microbiologist, consultant, 106
    see also Chief Pathologist
Midwives, subject to medical prescrip-
        tion, 125
Miles, A. W. et al, 64, 257
Miller, E. J. et al, 34, 38
Ministry of Health, Circular HM (60)
        45, 78
    Circular HM (61) 112, 78
    Circular HM (54) 109, 81
    Circular HM (55) 82, 81
    First Green Paper, 248
    Second Green Paper, 252
Monitoring and co-ordinating, 82, 86,
        95, 104, 173, 174, 176, 215
    by Chief Administrator, 173
    by Group Secretary, 174, 176
    functional, 62, 221
    in unified and multiple management,
        218
Monitoring role, 267
Mouzelis, N. P., 6, 69
Multiple management system, 218-20

N.H.S., 255
    Act 1946, 19, 26, 190, 197, 207, 208
    Central O and M Unit, 163
    Consultative Document on the
        Future, 218
    reorganization, 218
    structure, 14
Nadel, S. F., 36
National Council of Nurses, Joint
        Working Party, 146
National Health Service, see N.H.S.
Naylor, Maurice, 224
Newman, A. D. et al, 27, 63, 229, 277
Noel-Hall Report, 115

Non-operational roles, 38, 196, 247
North London Hospital Group, 2
North West Metropolitan Regional Hospital Board, 1, 40, 74, 119, 276
Northwick Park Hospital, 2
Nurse, questions explored with, 5
  role of, 121, 146, 140, 141
  training, relationship to nursing service, 140, 141
Nurses, charge, 129, 131, 134
  learner, 134
  relationship to, doctors, 124
    domestic staff, 162-9
Nursing hierarchy, 128, 136
  in small hospitals, special problems, 144, 145
  managerial and supervisory staff roles in, 132, 137
  and midwifery, 191, 193
  night organization, 139
  staff officer roles in, 134

OCCUPATIONAL, groups, 223, 230, 231, 232
  therapists, 100, 101
    relationship to nursing staff, 120, 123
  see also Paramedical staff
Operational, activities of the hospital service, 189-96
  and other activities, organizational division of, 246-9
  and other functions, 32
  services, providers of, 196
  work, 38
Ophthalmic opticians, 17
Ophthalmology, hierarchical organization of, 105
Opticians, 17
Organization, at Group and Hospital level, 153-6
  definition of, 34, 35
  objects of, 25
Organizational goals, 35, 36
Orthoptists, 101
Otolaryngology, 105
Outpatients department, 137, 138
Outposting, 60, 269
Owen, A. H., 253
Oxford, United Hospitals, Executive Committee, 246

PACKWOOD, G. F. L., 59
Paediatricians, see Consultant paediatricians
Pantall, J. et al, 4, 12
Paramedical, department, Consultants in, 109, 110
  staff, organization of, 100-18
Parsons, T., 79, 298
Pathology, complex, 106, 107
  Consultant in, 86, 87
  organization of, 107
Patient, and doctor, 79, 80
  treatment of, 224, 226
Perrow, C., 13, 34, 73, 96
Personnel, officer roles, 57
  resources, provision of, 247
Pharmacists, 16, 100, 113-18
Pharmacy, Noel-Hall Report, 115
  organization of, 153-6
Physical medicine, 105, 108, 109
Physical-superintendent role of, 83, 84
Physicist, chief, 86
Physicists, 101, 107, 114
Physiotherapist, Superintendent, 9 ,
  100, 101, 115, 120
  see also Paramedical staff
Platt Report, 98
Policy, definition of, 269
Popper, K. R., 294
Porters, 120, 149, 151, 169, 177
Principal Nursing Officer, 120, 129, 131, 134, 135, 136, 137, 138, 140, 141, 142, 143
Profession, 78, 79, 96, 97
  and professionalization, 97, 98
Professional, and semi-professional, 96
  autonomy, 214-8
  training, 231
Psychiatric, cases, integration of services for, 227
  nursing, 126
  Social Worker, 114
Psychiatrist, treatment prescribing authority of, 126
Psychologists, clinical, 114
Pugh, D. S. et al, 296

RADCLIFFE-BROWNE, 298
Radiographers, 101, 105, 106, 110, 111, 112
Radiologists, 86, 106, 108, 109, 110

Ranks and grades, 130, 131, 220, 221, 270
Reader, L. G., 13, 226
Reception services, 173
Reddin, W. T., 67
Redhill and Netherne Group, 1
Regional, Architect, 19
  Headquarters Nursing Staff, 284
  Health Authoriy, 51
  Hospital Board and H.M.C., 199-209
  Hospital Board Chief Officers, 233
  Nursing Officer, 19, 202, 203, 284
  Secretary, 19
  Specialists, 148
  Treasurer, 19
Representative, 198-200, 229-61
  role, 63, 64, 94, 270
  systems, 68, 278
Requisite organization, 4, 6, 35, 42, 280, 297, 298, 299
Research and teaching, see Clinical research and teaching
  conferences, 282
Revans, R. W., 4, 7, 12, 67, 132, 286, 289
Review and grievance systems, 257, 258
Richardson, R., 37
Roethlisberger, F. J. et al, 6
Roles, operational and non-operational, 32, 33
  production control and programming, 77
  production engineering, 57
Rowbottom, R. et al, 114, 216
Royal College of Nursing, Joint Report, 146

SALMON REPORT, 13, 33, 56, 119, 120, 127, 129, 130, 132, 134, 137, 138, 146, 148, 164, 166, 206
Scientific approach, characteristics of, 294, 295
Scottish Group Medical Superintendent, actual duties of, 238
Secondment, 62, 162, 221, 231, 271, 272
Secretary of State, 18, 21, 81
Seebohm Report, 18
Semi-professions, 231
Senior Administrative Medical Officer, 81
Service, giver, 55
  relationships, 52-6, 272

Sheffield Regional Hospital Board, Secretary to, 223, 224
Silverman, D., 34, 67, 298
Simon, H. A., 256
Sleight, P. et al, 246
Small hospitals, special problems of nursing, 144
Smith, H. L., 13, 73, 85
Social, analysis, 276-300
  Services, 253
    Departments, 18
  Organization Research Unit (Brunel), 213
  workers, 216
    medical, see Medical social workers
Sofer, C., 299
Speech therapists, role, 101, 114
Staff, committees, 278
  Officer, 56-9
    roles in nursing, 134-6
  relationship, 273
Staines Group, 2
Stanton, A. N. et al, 6
Statutory bodies, non-representative nature of at present, 222
Steering committees, 3
Stewart, R., 209
Stinchcombe, A. L., 35
Stuart-Clark, A. C., 197
Student nurse, 141
Subordinate relationship, 42-5, 51, 52, 68, 87, 273
Superior-subordinate relationship, 200
Supervisory, relationship, 46, 274
  roles, 133-4, 150
Supplies, 122, 149, 161, 162
  officer, 54, 148
  organization, Hut Report on, 161, 162
  specialists, 100
  staff, organization of, 149, 152

TEACHING STAFF (nursing), 141, 143
Technicians, 105, 106, 107
Telephone services, 169
Telephonists, organization of, 149
Theatre, attendants, 196
  suite, 137
Time-span, of discretion, 37, 130
  measure, 170
Tolliday, H., 41
Toulmin, S., 294
Trainee nurses, 140, 141

Transport services, 173
Treasurer, role of, 182-7
    Group, 3, 20, 82, 184, 185, 186, 202, 203
    Regional, 202, 203
Treatment-prescribing relationship, 45, 46, 88, 89, 225, 275
Tripartite management, 100, 234
    and multiple-management system, 218-20

WARD, aides, 163
    housekeepers, *see* Domestic organization
    sisters, 52, 54, 84, 164, 165
    nurses, 126
Weiland, G. F. et al, 3, 4, 12, 286, 289, 299

Welsh Hospital Board, 18
Westminster Hospital, 1, 148
Whitley Council Circular (PTB 179), 152
Williams, D., 4
Wilson, 87
Woodbine-Parish Report, 148, 158
Woodward, J., 296
Working Relationships in the British Hospital Service, 41
Works organization, 158
    see also Engineering and building

X-RAY DEPARTMENT, organization of, 105, 106

ZUCKERMAN REPORT, 100

E 3